Bone and Joint Futures

Edited by
Anthony D Woolf

Duke of Cornwall Rheumatology Department,
Royal Cornwall Hospital, Truro, UK

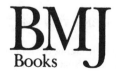

© BMJ Books 2002
BMJ Books is an imprint of the BMJ Publishing Group

First published in 2002
by BMJ Books, BMA House, Tavistock Square,
London WC1H 9JR

www.bmjbooks.com

British Library Cataloguing in Publication Data

A catalogue record for this book is available from the British Library

ISBN 0 7279 1548 7

Typeset by Newgen Imaging Systems (P) Ltd., Chennai
Printed and bound in Spain by GraphyCems, Navarra

Contents

Contributors

Ross A Benthien
Department of Orthopaedic Surgery, University of Connecticut Health Center, Connecticut, USA

Ferdinand C Breedveld
Department of Rheumatology, Leiden University Medical Centre, Leiden, Netherlands

Bruce D Browner
Gray-Gossling Professor and Chair, Department of Orthopaedic Surgery, University of Connecticut Health Center, Connecticut, USA

Juliet Compston
Department of Medicine, University of Cambridge School of Medicine, Addenbrooke's Hospital, Cambridge, UK

Peter Croft
Professor of Primary Care Epidemiology, Primary Care Sciences Research Centre, Keele University, UK

Michael Doherty
Professor of Rheumatology, University of Nottingham Medical School, UK

Stefan Lohmander
Professor of Orthopaedics, Department of Orthopaedics, University Hospital, Lund, Sweden

Donncha O'Gradaigh
Department of Medicine, University of Cambridge, School of Medicine, Cambridge, UK

Piet LCM van Riel
Department of Rheumatology, University Medical Centre Nijmegen, Nijmegen, Netherlands

Deborah PM Symmons
Professor of Rheumatology and Musculoskeletal Epidemiology, University of Manchester Medical School, Manchester, UK; Honorary Consultant Rheumatologist, East Cheshire NHS Trust, UK

Anthony D Woolf
Duke of Cornwall Rheumatology Department, Royal Cornwall Hospital, Truro, UK

Foreword

On January 13, 2000, the Bone and Joint Decade was formally launched at the headquarters of the World Health Organization in Geneva, Switzerland. This comes on the heels of the November 30, 1999 endorsement by the United Nations. UN Secretary General, Kofi Annan said, "There are effective ways to prevent and treat these disabling disorders, but we must act now. Joint diseases, back complaints, osteoporosis and limb trauma resulting from accidents have an enormous impact on individuals and societies, and on healthcare services and economies."

Musculoskeletal conditions are among the most common medical conditions with a substantial influence on health, quality of life and the use of resources. Medicine, more and more based on sophisticated technology, is becoming very expensive. At the same time the world population is ageing. The number of individuals over the age of 50 in the world is expected to double between 1990 and 2020. In Europe by 2010, for the first time, there will be more people over 60 years of age than less than 20 years, and by 2020 the elderly will represent 25% of the population, 100 million people.

The impact of musculoskeletal dieases is in a large part a function of its prevalence in the population. *Joint diseases* account for half of all chronic conditions in persons aged over 65. Some 25% of people over the age of 60 have significant pain and disability from joint diseases. The economic consequences are enormous – it is for example the first rated cause of work loss, in spite of being a condition that causes most problems to the population after retirement of age.

Back pain is the second leading cause of sick leave. *Low back pain* is the most frequent cause of limitation of activity in the young and middle aged, one of the most common reasons for medical consultation, and the most frequent occupational injury.

Musculoskeletal trauma accounts for about half of all reported injuries. It is anticipated that 25% of health expenditure of developing countries will be spent on trauma-related care by the year 2010 which is twice as much as the total loans given today.

Fragility fractures have doubled in the last decade. 40% of all women over 50 years will suffer from an osteoporotic fracture. The number of hip fractures will rise from about 1.7 million in 1990 to 6.3 million by 2050 unless aggressive preventive programs are started. However today evidence based prevention and treatment is available.

The selected contributions in this book, focusing on the future for bone and joint disorders in health policy, basic science and clinical development, will significantly help towards the aims of the Bone and Joint Decade.

L Lidgren
Chairman, The Bone and Joint Decade

For more information on the Bone and Joint Decade Strategies, visit:
www.boneandjointdecade.org

1: The future provision of care for musculoskeletal conditions

ANTHONY D WOOLF

What are the various musculoskeletal conditions?

Musculoskeletal conditions have an enormous and growing impact worldwide. Chronic musculoskeletal pain is reported in surveys by 1 in 4 people in both less and more developed countries. There is a wide spectrum of musculoskeletal conditions. Osteoarthritis, using disability-adjusted life-years, is the fourth most frequent predictive cause of problems worldwide in women and the eighth in men. Rheumatoid arthritis has a prevalence of 1–2% in women over 50 years and restricts work capacity in one third within the first year. Fractures related to osteoporosis will be sustained by approximately 40% of all Caucasian women over 50 years of age. The one year prevalence of low back pain in the UK is almost 50%. There are an estimated 23 million to 34 million people injured worldwide each year due to road traffic accidents. In addition, work related musculoskeletal disorders were responsible for 11 million days lost from work in 1995 in the UK. In the Swedish Cost of Illness Study, musculoskeletal conditions represented almost a quarter of the total cost of illness. Epidemiological studies in less developed countries show that musculoskeletal conditions are an equally important problem, as in the more developed countries. This burden is increasing throughout the world with population growth and the change in risk factors such as increased longevity, urbanisation and motorisation, particularly in the less developed countries.

What burden do they cause to individuals and to society?

Musculoskeletal conditions are characterised by pain and are usually associated with loss of function. Many are chronic or recurrent. They are the commonest cause of long term impairments reported in the USA. Chronic diseases are defined by the US Centres for Disease and Prevention as illnesses "that are prolonged, do not resolve spontaneously and are rarely cured completely" but the Long Term Medical Conditions Alliance has emphasised how they also impact on peoples' emotional and social well being; on their social, community and working lives; and on their relationships. The recently revised WHO International Classification of Functioning tries to capture more effectively the effect these conditions have on a person's quality of life. At the first level the condition may impair or result in the loss of specific functions. This will secondly affect the activities that the person can do. At the third level the condition can affect how the individual can function within society, their participation and the restrictions imposed upon that. Musculoskeletal conditions affect people at all levels. For example, a person with osteoarthritis of the knees will have an impairment of decreased movement and strength in both lower limbs (body function level). The person will be limited in the activity of moving around (person level functioning). In addition due to the fact that there are no lifts but many steps in the buildings in the person's environment, the person experiences much more difficulty with moving around and thus this person's real life performance is worse than the capacity he/she possesses (societal level functioning): a clear restriction of participation imposed by the environment of that person. It may prevent them from working and result in loss of independence. The effect any condition has on an individual will also be dependent on many contextual factors, both personal and environmental – housing, carer support, financial situation, the person's beliefs and expectations. The importance of these must also be recognised. The impact is restricted not just to the individual, but it can also affect the family and carers.

Many people with musculoskeletal conditions can no longer fully contribute to society and require support that may be chronic depending on the nature of the condition. As a consequence musculoskeletal conditions have a major socioeconomic impact in terms of days off work, dependency on carers, social security payments and the other aspects of indirect costs of illness. In the Swedish Cost of Illness Study the majority of the costs were indirect relating to this morbidity and disability.

What are the healthcare needs?

The broad impact of any chronic disease must be considered when assessing needs and how best to meet them. The pervasive nature of most musculoskeletal conditions means they have a major impact on all aspects of quality of life, not just aspects of health related quality of life. However, the future provision of health care must initially concentrate on health related aspects but society should recognise and allow for these broader effects of chronic disease. There are several important issues for people with long term conditions. They have a close relationship with clinicians and this must be based on mutual trust and respect. They increasingly want to be responsible consumers of health care if the providers of that care create an environment in which patients can receive guidance. They need to form partnerships with healthcare professionals for their long term care. Clinicians must be aware that they only experience for a few moments in time the problems that any individual with a chronic musculoskeletal condition is trying to cope with every day. It is important to improve quality of life even where there is no cure, to give support and to ensure the person fulfils his/her life as much as is achievable within the constraints imposed by the condition. It is essential to focus on the individual *with* the long term condition and not just view the individual *as* the long term condition. There is therefore a focus on care and support for many of these conditions in contrast to cure, although this may well change in the future with advances in treatment. What is achievable has already changed dramatically over the last decade.

The WHO approach for identifying the impact of a condition can also identify specific needs – a clinician or a rehabilitation therapist might be concerned with the impairment or capacity/activity limitations, while consumer organisations and activists might be concerned with participation problems. Thinking in terms of limitations of function, activities and participation provides a common language that enables one to identify what can be done for the person and what can be done for the person's environment to enhance his or her independence and to measure the effects of these interventions.

The needs of the individual with a chronic musculoskeletal condition may not just be health related, as environmental factors such as availability of transportation, access to buildings, or social factors such as availability of appropriate local employment, are equally important in achieving quality of life. Health care will not meet such needs now or in the future but there are other ways in which society can respond to these needs through social support and policy. However, the clinician has the important role of advocacy on behalf of people with these needs.

In addition to these principal needs there are the specific needs of the condition that must be met – relieving the symptoms and preventing progression where cure is not possible. There must be appropriate healthcare services for these needs.

What are the goals of management?

Musculoskeletal conditions are painful, mostly chronic, often progressive with structural damage and deformity and associated with loss of function. Specific functions are impaired, and this restricts personal activities and limits participation in society. The reputation of arthritis and other musculoskeletal conditions is well known so that their onset is associated with fear of loss of independence. The aims of management are prevention where possible and effective treatment and rehabilitation for those who already have these conditions.

There are therefore different goals for different players. The public health goal is to maximise the health of the population and central to this are preventative strategies that target the whole population, such as increasing the levels of physical activity or reducing obesity. However, it is very difficult to change people's lifestyles – the risks of smoking are widely known yet it is an increasingly common activity amongst younger people. Targeting high risk individuals is another approach providing there are recognised risk factors of sufficient specificity and acceptable interventions that can be used to reduce risk once identified.

The management of people with musculoskeletal conditions has much more personalised goals. They want to know what it is – what is the diagnosis and prognosis. They want to know what will happen in the future and they therefore need education and support. They want to know how to help themselves and the importance of self-management is increasingly recognised. They want to know how they can do more and they need help to reduce the functional impact. Importantly they need to be able to control their pain effectively. They also wish to prevent the problem from progressing and require access to the effective treatments that are increasingly available.

This requires the person with a musculoskeletal condition to be informed and empowered and supported by an integrated multidisciplinary team that has the competencies and resources to achieve the goals of management. The person should be an active member of that team, and it is his or her condition and associated problems that should be the subject of the team.

What can be done – the present situation and current issues

There have been dramatic changes in the last decade affecting what can be achieved in the management of musculoskeletal conditions, but for various reasons these benefits are not reaching all those who could profit.

The current provision of care for musculoskeletal conditions reflects the past and current priorities given to these common but chronic and largely incurable conditions. The high prevalence of these conditions, many of which do not require complex procedures or techniques to treat effectively, and the lack of specialists means that most care is provided in the community by the primary care team. This contrasts with the lack of expertise in the management of musculoskeletal conditions in primary care, since undergraduate education in orthopaedics and rheumatology is minimal in many courses and few doctors gain additional experience whilst in training for primary care. In addition there is little training in the principles of management of patients with chronic disease when understanding and support are so important in the current absence of the effective interventions we would like to offer. The increased prevalence with age results in an attitude that these problems are inevitable. The consequence of these factors is that the patient all too often gets the impression that they should "put up and shut up", "learn to live with it" because "it is to be expected" as part of their age. Although developing coping skills is an essential part of managing to live despite having a chronic disease, it is a positive approach and not one of dismissal. A greater understanding by all clinicians, particularly in primary care, of the impact of musculoskeletal conditions and how to manage them is essential to attain the outcomes which are currently achievable by best clinical practice.

Secondary care is largely based on the historical development of the relevant specialities rather than by planning. Orthopaedics has largely evolved from trauma services but has undergone dramatic developments in the past 40 years with the development of arthroplasties. Rheumatology has evolved from the backgrounds of spa therapy and internal medicine. Physical therapy and rehabilitation has strong links with the armed forces. Manual medicine has developed to meet the demand of soft tissue musculoskeletal conditions and back pain. The growth of alternative and complementary therapies reflects the failure of interventions to meet

5

the patient's expectations and the large numbers with chronic musculoskeletal conditions seeking a more effective and better tolerated, more natural intervention. The development of pain clinics and services for helping people cope with chronic pain reflect ways of trying to help people manage the predominant symptom of musculoskeletal conditions.

Secondary specialist care is within the hospital sector in the UK but predominantly outpatient based, and inpatient beds have often been in the smaller older hospitals that provided the subacute or rehabilitation services – caring more than curative interventions. There has been a trend over several decades for these smaller units to close and services to be concentrated in larger district general hospitals where there is enormous competition for the ever reducing numbers of beds for inpatient care. Many rheumatologists now train with little experience of inpatient facilities and therefore, for example, have little experience of what can be achieved by intensive rehabilitation alongside intensive drug therapy to control inflammatory joint disease. Lack of hospital facilities is now causing difficulties with the parenteral administration of newer biological therapies.

The management of musculoskeletal conditions is multidisciplinary but the integration of the different musculoskeletal specialities varies between centres. Usually rheumatologists or orthopaedic surgeons work closely with the therapists but there is little integration of the medical specialities themselves and there are few examples of clinical departments of musculoskeletal conditions embracing orthopaedics, rheumatology, rehabilitation, physiotherapy and occupational therapy, supported by specialist nurses, orthotics, podiatry, dietetics and all the other relevant disciplines. Hopefully this will change with time as part of the integrated activites of the "Bone and Joint Decade".

The outcome of musculoskeletal conditions has altered greatly. For many musculoskeletal conditions there are now effective strategies for prevention, treatments to control or reverse the disease processes and methods of rehabilitation to minimise impact and allow people to achieve their potential. This is detailed in subsequent chapters but some examples are given. Trauma can be prevented in many circumstances such as road traffic accidents, land mines and in the workplace if the effective policies are implemented. The management of trauma can now result in far less long term disability if appropriate services are available in a timely and appropriate fashion. It is possible to identify those at risk of osteoporosis and target treatment to prevent fracture. Treatment can also prevent the progression of osteoporosis even after the first fracture, with drugs which maintain or even increase bone strength. Structural changes can be prevented in rheumatoid arthritis by effective second line therapy with recognition of the need for early diagnosis and intervention. Osteoarthritis cannot yet be prevented but large joint arthroplasty has dramatically altered the impact that it has on ageing individuals who would have lost their independence. There have been major developments in preventing back pain becoming chronic. There have been major advances in the management of pain. Pain control can now be much more effectively achieved with new ranges of effective and well tolerated drugs, and there have been advances in techniques related to a greater understanding of the mechanisms of pain and its chronification.

There remain many outstanding problems concerning the management of musculoskeletal conditions. There are many interventions in use for which there is little evidence to prove effectiveness. Many of these are complex interventions dependent on the therapist, such as physiotherapy, or provision of social support and these are complex to evaluate. Evidence is, however, essential to ensure such interventions, if truly effective, are adequately resourced in the future.

Many, however, are not benefiting from the proven advances and achieving the potentially improved outcomes. This is largely because of lack of awareness, resources and priority. These resources are not just money to pay for new expensive drugs but also the human resources of clinicians and therapists with the necessary competencies to effectively manage those with musculoskeletal conditions. The public and many health professionals are not fully aware of what can now be achieved and therefore perpetuate a negative attitude. If they think little can be done, they do not seek expert help. Lack of awareness and knowledge of medical advances means that these are not delivered to the main benefactor – the patient. There are many suffering pain which could be much more effectively managed. Many have impaired function inappropriately. Lack of knowledge of what can be achieved alongside a lack of awareness of the enormous burden on the individual and society leads to lack of priority and resources. There are few health policies that highlight the importance of musculoskeletal conditions despite their enormous costs to society and to the individual. As a consequence, for example, the waiting times for joint replacement surgery for osteoarthritis, a highly cost effective intervention, are amongst the longest in the UK.

The challenge is to ensure as many people as possible can benefit from the current effective means of prevention, treatment and rehabilitation.

What is the future

Demand

The demand for care for musculoskeletal conditions is going to increase. The global disease burden of non-communicable diseases was 36% in 1990 but it is predicted to be 57% in 2020. There are several reasons. First, because of the change in population demographics. By 2030, 25% of the population in the UK will be over the age of 65 years and the prevalence of musculoskeletal conditions increases dramatically with age. Lifestyle changes that have happened in westernised countries are likely to increase musculoskeletal conditions, but most worryingly these lifestyle changes are also happening in the developing world along with inversion of the age pyramid which will result in the greatest predicted growth in chronic diseases. Lack of exercise will not only increase cardiovascular disease but exercise is also important in the prevention of osteoarthritis, maintaining bone mass and preventing falls. However, surveys in Sweden have shown that about 25–30% of middle aged men and 10–15% of middle aged women are completely inactive. It is also estimated that only 20% of the population who are 30 years and older are, from a health standpoint and when regarding physical conditions, sufficiently physically active. This means that almost 80% of the adult population in Sweden over the age of 30 is either not adequately physically active or completely inactive. Other risk factors for musculoskeletal conditions that show similarly unfavourable trends are motorisation with subsequent accidents, obesity, smoking and excess alcohol.

Demand also relates to the expectation for health and this is increasing. At present many suffer in silence outside the healthcare system because they feel that little can be done for them. Many primary care doctors do not seek the latest interventions for their patients because of lack of awareness of what can be achieved. However, as there is increasing awareness of what is achievable, so there will be increasing demand. New technologies generate this demand and also contribute to the increased costs. In addition as the expectation of the right to good health related quality of life increases, then those in developing countries who, for example, are currently suffering back pain silently will increasingly identify it as a health problem and expect medical intervention and social support.

Provision of health care

The way in which health care is provided can affect the level of care delivered and its outcome and this is the focus of current activity by WHO (World Health Organization). At present equal levels of care are not being delivered as there are countries of similar levels of income, education, industrial attainment and health expenditure with a wide variety of health outcomes. Some of this is due to differences in performance of the health systems. A health system includes all the activities whose primary purpose is to promote, restore or maintain health and can therefore even include efforts to improve road safety where the primary intention is to reduce road traffic accidents (WHO World Health Report 2000). The health of the population should reflect the health of individuals throughout life and include both premature mortality and non-fatal health outcomes as key components. A health system should also be responsive to the legitimate expectations of the population such as respecting their dignity, confidentiality and involving them in decisions. There should also be fairness in financial contribution so that households should not become impoverished or pay an excessive share of income for healthcare and poor households should pay less than rich. Obviously the performance of any healthcare system can only be measured in relation to the resources available. The WHO World Health Report will now give information each year on the performance of health systems of each country within this framework.

This failure of many health systems along with rising demands for health care, rising costs and limited resources is generating much debate about the most effective systems for the provision of health care. Economic and social development in all countries is increasingly taking a "market approach" and health can be viewed as another commodity. This must be balanced against the recognition that good health is a prerequisite for human development and for maintaining peace and security. It is also important that any system is equitable for all diseases whether acute and treatable or chronic disorders that require more care and support. Musculoskeletal conditions, as a major contributor to such non-fatal outcomes, need greater recognition of their importance and their specific needs must be considered to ensure appropriate systems of care.

There is a movement towards managing care so that the healthcare system provides cost-effective health care within the available resources. Managed care has developed in the USA where an organisation assumes responsibility for all necessary health care for an individual in exchange for fixed payment. Socialised healthcare systems in the UK and Sweden are also systems that provide this form of care. This approach may not be the ideal for all countries but the tools of managed care may be of relevance. The three tools are first to be able to manage demand, secondly to have some control over management and finally to be able to influence care delivery so that it is cost effective. Demand can be controlled by making payments based on capitation not clinical activity, introducing gatekeepers to expensive secondary care, making some direct costs to the user and educating the public so that they are better able to care for themselves. Although some of these may be feared as barriers to professional and patient freedom of choice, making the person with the condition a more informed user of health care is in keeping with the principles of chronic disease management. Control over medical management is potentially more restrictive of clinical freedom but something many physicians are already used to where permission is required from the funder before certain interventions can be performed. The use of evidence-based guidelines is also increasing and a principal of healthcare reforms in the UK. The important changes in the delivery of care are the increasing access of the public to advice through telemedicine and promoting self-care with greater use of non-doctors. This may be more appropriate to chronic diseases providing that it achieves the same outcome as more expert care, and that this outcome is measured for all the goals of managing people with musculoskeletal conditions. These changes represent a reversal from "industrial age medicine" in which professional care dominates to "information age healthcare" in which professional care provides support to a system that emphasises self-care. Healthcare providers will progress from managing disease to promoting health. Lifetime plans for health promotion will be built on an intimate knowledge of the person and their risk factors for various conditions.

Within this context of changing systems of health care are the implications of how it will be delivered. What will be the resources in human capital as well as physical? What will be the political priorities?

The settings for health care have changed over the centuries with the changes in what is expected and developments in what can be done. Hospitals have played a dominant role in the provision of care, and they have evolved during the twentieth century from institutions that provide basic care and support to settings for medical treatment of increasing sophistication, effectiveness and cost. Advances in diagnosis have lead to the recognition of new, often treatable diseases. This has been paralleled by the massive expansion in pharmaceuticals. There have been enormous changes in what can be achieved. Infectious diseases are becoming less common and interventions are meaning that many chronic incurable diseases are now becoming treatable and controllable, such as peptic ulcer disease, childhood leukaemias, some solid cancers, transplantation and now the treatment of rheumatoid arthritis and osteoporosis. There are now two competing roles for hospitals – highly technical procedure and "cure" based centres and, by contrast, centres that provide care which is usually multidisciplinary therapist based. The changes in systems of health care mean that such specialist facilities, although likely to remain a key part in the management of acute and chronic diseases, will increasingly be just one part of the infrastructure to effectively prevent and treat musculoskeletal conditions. Provision of care closer to the person with the problem and more designed to help them manage their own health will need to be developed. The trends to develop skilled multidisciplinary teams that cross the various health sectors, to develop specialist nurses as key members of such teams as well as improving access to expert information and advice using technology will meet many of these aims and reduce demands on specialist medical services. Specialised services will continue to have a major role in facilitating care, developing evidence-based strategies, undertaking research, providing education for the healthcare team as well as for those with musculoskeletal conditions, and directly managing more complex cases. Their role is likely to become more strategic rather than just "hands on".

Management

There are also future trends in the management of musculoskeletal conditions. More priority will be given to implementing primary prevention in response to the growing health and social demands of these conditions, and looking at the health of the population and not just of the individual. Consumers are assuming more responsibility for their own health and also in planning and providing services and monitoring and evaluating their outcomes. Self-management has been demonstrated to be an effective component of the management of those with chronic conditions. The preferences of the individual will need to be increasingly considered in planning their management and clinicians will have to facilitate this as well as provide treatment. A greater level of understanding of health by the public will be necessary for this to work. The effective use of consumer health informatics is also central to this and the rapid technological developments mean that the person will be increasingly able to meet their individual information needs. Ensuring the quality and appropriateness of this information will be the challenge.

There are also going to be major changes in the future about what can actually be achieved through advances from research. It may become possible to prevent diseases such as rheumatoid arthritis once the trigger is identified. There are also various attempts at tissue repair using either tissue transplants or growth factors. Autologous chondrocyte transplantation is being used to repair articular cartilage defects and bone morphogenic proteins and transforming growth factor beta to enhance fracture healing. Gene therapy may be a future way of delivering such growth factors. New materials are being used for surgical implantation which may make it an option for the middle aged and not just for the elderly person. The skills to revise large joint arthroplasty are sophisticated but continuing developments are likely to prolong the life of a prosthesis and ensure the lifelong restoration of function to the damaged joint. The development of anti-tumour necrosis factor alpha (anti-TNF-α) has demonstrated how a clear understanding of pathogenesis can lead to an effective targeted intervention that can control disease and prevent tissue damage. There is also evidence that the early diagnosis and treatment of rheumatoid arthritis results in better outcomes. If diseases can be put into prolonged remission we will be able to talk of cure. The ability to put many forms of cancer into long term remission has totally altered attitudes and priorities to cancer, and it is now a priority to diagnose and treat cancer as early as possible. The enormous investments into different approaches to effectively modify, if not cure, chronic progressive diseases is likely to pay off during the next few decades. There must be an increased ability to identify those with these conditions as soon as possible before tissue damage is irreversible and effective interventions initiated.

It is increasingly clear that the delivery of high quality of care depends on an improved evidence base to clinical practice with systems of quality assurance and this is rapidly developing in the UK. This, alongside the setting of targets and outcome indicators, guarantees a high quality of care. This approach also leads to cost containment. These trends are therefore likely to continue. At present much of the management of musculoskeletal conditions has a small evidence base and many of the indicators that are currently used by the WHO and UK government to monitor health have limited relevance to musculoskeletal conditions. There is an urgent need for research to clarify which interventions are cost effective, to develop strategies for their implementation and establish indicators that better reflect the burden of musculoskeletal conditions and can monitor the effectiveness of interventions. The development of electronic health records will increase the value of having valid indicators to audit care. All those involved in the management of musculoskeletal conditions must actively become involved in this process so that they remain active partners in the effective management of these conditions.

In the next 20 years there are clearly going to be enormous changes in demand for more effective management of musculoskeletal conditions; advances in what can be achieved, which may move some of the conditions away from being identified as chronic and incurable to diseases which are recognised as treatable if identified early; and also changes in systems of care, which may or may not be of advantage to the management of musculoskeletal conditions.

What is the ideal model of care for musculoskeletal conditions?

The characteristics of musculoskeletal conditions and key principles of their care have been discussed. Prevention may reduce the numbers with or severity of musculoskeletal conditions but we now need to consider the ideal model for the care of these conditions when chronic or recurrent, which have a pervasive impact on the person's quality of life as well as affecting their families and friends.

Community

The community plays an important role in supporting care for chronically ill patients. People with musculoskeletal conditions, even if requiring intensive medical care, spend most of their time within the community and that is where support is needed. Apart from general understanding and support, gained through a greater awareness of musculoskeletal conditions and their impacts, the community can help through providing specific facilities, such as for exercise, and ensure that the local environment does not create barriers for those less physically able. Support groups for those with chronic disease provide valuable help and encouragement. They can provide more specific help, such as by giving information, ensuring the person gains appropriate help within the social welfare system or promoting and teaching self-management.

The broader community also plays a critical role in setting health and social policies – ensuring the provision of appropriate services, insurance benefits, civil rights laws for persons with disabilities and other health-related regulations that affect the lives of people with a chronic condition. They have a powerful voice in any democracy.

Health system

A system seeking to improve the health of those with musculoskeletal conditions must ensure the focus of care is not just for the acute episodes or those with systemic complications that can threaten life, but also delivers high quality care achieving the highest attainable outcomes by looking at the problems people have in their homes and communities as well as their problems with their personal health throughout the natural history of their condition. The system should not treat people differently dependent on the nature of the disorder they have – whether it is acute, chronic, curable, treatable or where symptom relief is the only option – neither should age related conditions be discriminated against because they are "inevitable". All should have access to high standards of care. However, private health insurers, in particular where there is an alternative system of care such as in the UK, are increasingly excluding chronic disease from their cover, which is of no help to the individual who does not choose one form of illness over another. Such discrimination is inappropriate. It is hoped that the new effective means of treating these conditions will in part counteract this attitude.

Ways of controlling demand should not unfairly affect those with musculoskeletal conditions. The gatekeeper should be competent to give the appropriate level of care and be able to recognise his/her limitations and know when a higher level of care can result in an improved outcome to avoid the rationalisation of care becoming the rationing of care. This requires higher levels of competency in the management of musculoskeletal conditions by the primary care team than presently exists. Support by an integrated multidisciplinary expert team that crosses the health sectors from secondary to primary care can also ensure cost effective management using an appropriate level of skill and intervention. Overtreatment is just as harmful as undertreatment in chronic musculoskeletal conditions, inducing dependency on healthcare interventions and expectation that cannot be fulfilled.

Self-management

People with musculoskeletal conditions must take better care of themselves and actively participate in their care to minimise the impact of their condition. They need to be trained in proven methods of minimising symptoms, impact and complications. However, effective self-management means more than telling patients what to do. It means giving patients a central role in determining their care, one that fosters a sense of responsibility for their own health. Using a collaborative approach, providers and patients must work together to define problems, set priorities, establish goals, create treatment plans and solve problems along the way. The multidisciplinary team must include the person with the musculoskeletal condition as a member of the team and not as its subject. Likewise the person must take responsibility and actively work towards helping themselves – not just receiving care but participating by, for example, doing exercise and losing weight if so advised. This approach will require the right attitudes by both the person with the musculoskeletal condition and by the providers of care as well as the means to provide education and support. Health consumer informatics has great potential to help with this, but it is the responsibility of the healthcare team to ensure the person understands the nature of his or her condition, what to expect and how to manage it. This requires an accurate diagnosis and then good communication and support. The latter should be given by all members of the team but the specialist nurse can play a vital role as they have the expertise and the ear of the patient who is frequently not receptive to information in the classic healthcare environment.

Delivery system

Improving the health of people with chronic conditions requires transforming a system that is essentially reactive, responding mainly when a person is sick due to an exacerbation or complication, to one that is proactive and focused on keeping a person as healthy and independent as possible. That requires not only determining what care is needed, but also spelling out roles and tasks and setting targets to ensure the patient gets the care – not just knowing a patient with rheumatoid arthritis needs monitoring of disease activity, but developing a system that ensures it happens. Audit should be used to ensure these systems are working and delivering the expected results. It requires making sure that all the providers who take care of a patient have up to date information about the patient's status. It also requires making follow-up a part of standard procedure, so patients are not only supported throughout their condition but also that their disease is monitored to facilitate optimal control within the current therapeutic options.

Decision support

Treatment decisions need to be based on explicit, proven guidelines supported by at least one defining study. These guidelines should be discussed with patients, so they can understand the principles behind their care. Those who make treatment decisions need ongoing training to remain up to date on the latest methods. Decision support also means keeping all members of the team fully informed of any treatment decisions and of the evidence base behind them.

Clinical information system

Effective care of any chronic condition is virtually impossible without information systems that track individual patients as well as populations of patients. The use of anti-TNF-α is resulting in the development of registers for rheumatoid arthritis but these are rudimentary or non-existent for most musculoskeletal conditions. Electronic health records will, as they are developed, help facilitate this. A system could check an individual's treatment to make sure it conforms to recommended guidelines, measure outcomes and help ensure the ideal control of his or her condition.

What resources are needed?

The provision of the ideal future care of musculoskeletal conditions will clearly need greater resources. It will be information lead and both public and healthcare professionals will require better awareness and knowledge. There needs to be easier public access to high quality unbiased information about musculoskeletal conditions and their management. All health professionals need a higher level of minimum competency in the diagnosis and management of musculoskeletal conditions. Minimum competencies in the management of musculoskeletal conditions are being established for all medical students by the Bone and Joint Decade Education Task Force. Standards for rheumatology training at the levels of undergraduate, specialist training and continuing professional development have already been established in Europe. Standards in primary care need raising through education and there is a diploma course available in the UK.

The multidisciplinary team needs the correct skill mix so that the medical, physical, functional, psychological, social and educational needs of the person with the musculoskeletal condition can be met. Each of these will need the appropriate competencies for managing musculoskeletal conditions. There needs to be sufficient numbers of such skilled individuals to ensure fair access to care. Fair access to proven cost effective interventions is also required, such as large joint arthroplasty or anti-TNF-α, and guidelines will be required to control and monitor this.

Research is required to develop more effective interventions and evidence must be provided of the effectiveness of any intervention to improve health. At present there is no relationship between research spending on musculoskeletal conditions compared to the costs of the problem. More investment is clearly required to reduce the burden of these common chronic diseases.

Obtaining more resources requires greater priority and political will. The enormous burden of these conditions is increasingly recognised and the Bone and Joint Decade initiative is raising awareness of what can and should be done to reduce this burden. At present, however, musculoskeletal conditions are a priority in only a few countries.

What are the barriers to change and achieving outcomes?

Although there are compelling reasons to improve the standards of care, there are clearly several obstacles. The argument is accepted that the burden will increase but the strategies to reduce this are not proven. Specific interventions have been shown to help individuals but there is little evidence for the effectiveness of strategies of care. It will remain difficult to gain the resources for major initiatives without appropriate evidence. It will be difficult to achieve the goals of improved health outcomes without the resources that have been identified.

Providing access to appropriate services, developing new services and introducing new treatments always has a cost even if it can be set against a distant future health gain. Strong business cases will have to be developed to compete effectively for funds.

Competing priorities within limited resources and knowledge of the potential costs of providing readily available care for these common conditions are the greatest barriers. The demonstration of the impact of musculoskeletal conditions on the individual and society using generic indicators will allow direct comparison to other conditions and will enable more appropriate priorities to be set. It is important in this context to consider musculoskeletal conditions as a whole, in the same way that mental illnesses or cancers have been considered together, when trying to establish broad areas of priority. Evidence however is much more effective if it is actively promoted and the Bone and Joint Decade initiative links professional and patient organisations and combines evidence with advocacy. It is hoped that this will help facilitate the future provision of appropriate care for musculoskeletal conditions.

Recommended reading

Calkins E, Boult C, Wanger EH, Pacala J. *New Ways to Care for Older People: Building Systems Based on Evidence*. New York: Springer, 1999.

Greenlick MR. The emergence of population-based medicine. *HMO Practice* 1995;**9**:120–2.

Institute for Health & Aging: University of California, San Francisco, for the Robert Wood Johnson Foundation. *Chronic care in America: A 21st century challenge*. San Francisco: Institute for Health & Aging, 1996.

Smith R. The future of healthcare systems. *BMJ* 1997;**314**:1495–6.

Wilson J. Acknowledging the expertise of patients and their organisations. *BMJ* 1999;**319**:771–4.

2: The future burden of bone and joint conditions; and priorities for health care

DEBORAH PM SYMMONS

Introduction

The natural watershed provided by a new century and a new millennium offers the opportunity not only to look back and contemplate the achievements of the last 100 years, but also to look forward and anticipate the challenges of the next. In the early part of the last century the major threat to the public's health was posed by infectious diseases. This remains the case in the developing world. In more developed countries the threat of infectious disease has been superseded by that of cardiovascular disease and cancer. There are now prospects for reducing the occurrence and improving the outcome of both cancer and heart disease. But treatments do not save lives – they postpone deaths. As life expectancy increases it becomes clear that there are new spectres waiting to impair health. Most musculoskeletal disorders increase in prevalence with advancing age and are destined to represent a major burden on public health in the next few decades. This chapter looks at projections for population growth and examines the implications of these demographic changes on the burden of some of the principal musculoskeletal disorders: rheumatoid arthritis (RA), osteoarthritis (OA), osteoporosis and back pain. It also considers whether there is any evidence of secular changes in the occurrence or outcome of these conditions.

The Global Burden of Disease Project

Each year the World Bank commissions a report on some aspect of economic development. In 1993, for the first time, it chose to focus on health. The report was called "Investing in Health" and it examined the interplay between human health, health policy and economic development.[1] The team that authored the report requested an assessment of the global burden of disease. The Global Burden of Disease Project was lead by Christopher Murray of Harvard University and Alan Lopez of the World Health Organization (WHO). They assembled a team of experts to assess the burden of disease by cause for eight regions predetermined by the World Bank (Box 2.1). The "burden" was quantified by combining measures of

---

Box 2.1 World Bank "Regions" 1993

- Established market economies
- Former Socialist countries
- Latin America and the Caribbean
- Middle Eastern Crescent
- Sub-Saharan Africa
- India
- China
- Other Asia and Islands

---

mortality and disability into a new measure called the disability-adjusted life year.[2] The experts assisted in modelling the number of cases, the case fatality rate and the associated disability for each condition; age and gender band; and region. Mortality estimates were based on chapters of the "International Classification of Diseases"[3] and so include all musculoskeletal conditions. Because of the limited time available to complete the report, only three musculoskeletal conditions could be included in the estimates of disability-adjusted life years: RA, osteoarthritis of the hip and osteoarthritis of the knee. All estimates were based on 1990 data. Figure 2.1 shows the mortality due to all musculoskeletal disorders for each of the eight World Bank regions. The greatest proportion of deaths due to musculoskeletal disorders was in the established market economies. The greatest proportion of years lived with disability (8.2%) is also found in the established market economies (Figure 2.2). To a large extent, mortality and morbidity from musculoskeletal disorders are proportional to total life expectancy. By contrast, the greatest proportion of deaths due to road traffic accidents occurs in Latin America and the Caribbean (Figure 2.3). The pattern shown in Figure 2.3 does not mirror either car ownership or regional wealth.

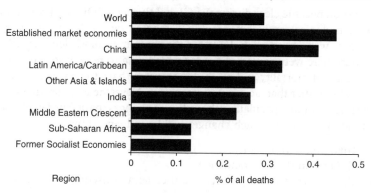

Figure 2.1   Mortality resulting from musculoskeletal conditions.

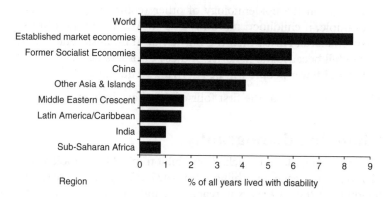

Figure 2.2   Years lived with disability resulting from musculoskeletal disorders.

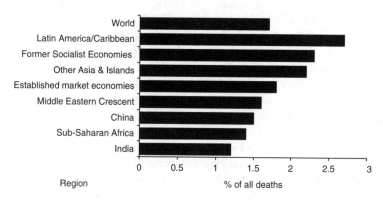

Figure 2.3   Mortality resulting from road traffic accidents.

It soon became clear during the Global Burden of Disease Project that epidemiological and demographic databases for many countries and diseases were quite weak. Even for the three musculoskeletal disorders chosen there were some regions for which data were very sparse. These estimates of mortality and morbidity therefore have to be viewed as best estimates rather than accurate assessments. Nevertheless, they do offer a starting point for speculating about future changes in the burden of bone and joint conditions. Such changes will be influenced by:

- changing demography
- changes in disease incidence
- changes in disease severity – either as a consequence of natural history or treatment
- changes in mortality due to the disease
- changes in the epidemiology of other (competing) disorders; for example, if childhood mortality due to AIDS continues to rise in sub-Saharan Africa then the burden of musculoskeletal disorders will fall because the majority of these disorders occur in late adult life and fewer people will be surviving to this age.

This chapter looks at the first four of the above influences.

Changing demography

The world population reached one billion in 1804. It took a further 123 years to reach two billion (in 1927), 33 years to reach three billion (in 1960), 14 years to reach four billion (in 1974), 13 years to reach five billion (in 1987) and 12 years to reach six billion on 12 October 1999.[4] The population is projected to grow still further so that by 2050 it will probably be around 8.9 billion (Figure 2.4). The structure of the population is likely to change dramatically especially in the more developed countries where, by 2050, it is anticipated that almost one quarter of the population will be aged more than 65 (Figure 2.5). Since most musculoskeletal disorders are more common in the elderly this has important implications for the number of cases particularly of arthritis and osteoporosis. Even if there is no change in the underlying age and sex specific incidence of these conditions, there will inevitably be a sharp rise in overall prevalence and therefore in the burden of disease. The changing structure of the population will also impact on the way that health care is funded. In 1950, in the more developed countries, 65% of the population were of working age whereas by 2050 only 59% will be in this age group (Figure 2.6). There will also

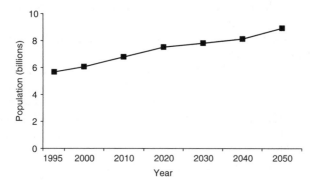

Figure 2.4 Projected change in the world population: 1950–2050.

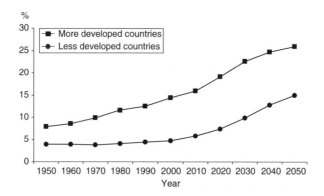

Figure 2.5 Proportion of total population aged over 65 years: 1950–2050.

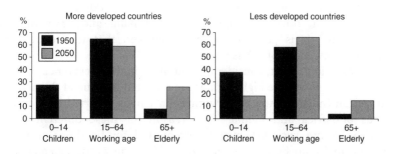

Figure 2.6 Population structures in more and less developed countries.

be a relative fall in the number of children and a rise in the very elderly who place greater demands on health services.

Europe is, and is projected to remain, the area of the world most affected by ageing. The proportion of the population aged over 60 is projected to rise from 20% in 1998 to 35% in 2050. Southern Europe is the oldest area with 22% aged over 60 in 1998, projected to rise to 39%. At present Italy has the greatest proportion of older people followed by Greece, Japan, Spain and Germany. By 2050 the country with the oldest population will be Spain. While European countries have the highest relative numbers (proportion) of older people, other regions have the highest absolute number. By 2050 three quarters of the world's elderly (aged over 65 years) population will live in Asia, Africa or Latin America. Growth of the elderly population is expected to plateau in North America, Europe and Russia by the second quarter of the twenty-first century but will continue to rise in Asia, Africa and Latin America. Nevertheless, by 2050 Africa will still have twice as many children as older people.

Rheumatoid arthritis

RA is the most common form of inflammatory joint disease worldwide. It has therefore been chosen as the index condition from this family. However, there are areas where this generalisation does not hold true; for example, among the people of the Polynesian Islands gout is far more common than RA.

Changes in disease occurrence

The cause of RA is unknown. The current view is that RA occurs as the result of exposure of a genetically susceptible individual to one or more of a variety of environmental triggers. A wide variety of potential environmental triggers has been identified including infections, immunisation, breast feeding, obesity, smoking and prior blood transfusion.[5] It is generally agreed, however, that the scope for primary prevention of RA is poor.[6]

There is, at present, considerable variation in the occurrence of RA around the globe. The highest rates are reported in some of the native American Indian groups and low rates have been reported from rural areas of Africa and China.[7] The reason for these differences is unclear. Some variation may be accounted for by differences in genetic make up between ethnic groups.[8] If this is the explanation then differences in RA occurrence are likely to persist. However, another suggested explanation is that RA is a "disease of civilisation". It was not convincingly described in Europe before 1800. In South Africa there is some suggestion that black Africans have a low rate of RA in rural areas but have the same rate as whites when they migrate to the city.[9] However, this same pattern was not seen in urban and rural areas amongst the Chinese – the prevalence of RA was low in both settings.[7,10] If some aspect of industrialised life acts as a trigger for RA then the occurrence in developing countries might be expected to rise.

There is some evidence that the incidence of RA amongst women has fallen in recent years in Europe[11] and the USA.[12] This has been attributed by some to the widespread use of the oral contraceptive pill, which is believed to offer some protection against the development of RA.[13] This protection may not be longlasting, however, and it may be that use of the oral contraceptive pill simply delays the onset of RA. There is direct evidence from Finland[14] and indirect evidence from review of publications on early RA that the median age of onset of RA is increasing. It is possible that there may be an increase in the frequency of late onset RA over the next couple of decades in the more developed countries as a consequence of widespread use of the oral contraceptive pill. It is difficult to predict what the impact of increased use of the oral contraceptive pill might be in developing countries where the incidence of RA is already low.

Whatever happens with regards to RA incidence, the prevalence is likely to rise quite steeply because of the demographic changes referred to above. In developing countries the median age of onset of RA is currently around 55 years.[14,15] Patients with RA are likely to benefit to some extent from the general improvement in life expectancy and, as new cases continue to occur in the older age groups, the overall number of cases is destined to increase.

Changes in disease course

There has been increasing emphasis in recent years on early aggressive treatment of RA. There is a considerable body of evidence that this improves the outcome of the disease in terms of disability[16] and probably mortality, certainly in the short term.[17] Whether this improved disease course can be maintained over the 20 or so years' duration of the disease is not yet clear. Most of the excess mortality in RA is related to comorbidity, in particular to coronary heart disease[18], and it is not clear whether improved disease control will influence this long-term outcome. The last year has seen the advent of a new second line agent[19] and the introduction of a new class of therapy – the biological agents.[20,21] It seems likely that the long-term outcome of RA can be further improved and the number of years lived with disability will fall – at least in those countries where these new therapies are affordable. However, even before the introduction of these new treatments, outcome had been improved with the use of methotrexate. Methotrexate is inexpensive and so may improve the outcome of patients in less affluent regions. Overall, therefore, it seems likely that the burden of disability, if not the burden of mortality, due to RA for the individual will fall.

In conclusion it is likely that the absolute number of RA cases worldwide will rise over the next few decades reflecting world population growth. The proportion of the world's population with RA will also rise, reflecting demographic changes in the age structure of the population. However, because of improved treatment, the impact of the disease on the individual will fall. It is difficult to predict how these two opposite trends in numbers and severity will interact with regards to the overall burden of RA.

Osteoarthritis

Osteoarthritis (OA) is the oldest disease known to have affected humankind. It is also currently one of the most common conditions, particularly in old age. OA occurring without apparent cause is referred to as "primary" OA, and when it follows an identifiable cause such as an injury, congenital abnormality, infection or inflammation affecting the joint it is termed "secondary" OA. OA occurs as a combination of two processes: cartilage breakdown and new bone (osteophyte) formation. The end result is often referred to as "joint failure" and is perhaps analogous to heart failure, renal failure and brain failure. OA may affect almost any joint. However, osteoarthritis of the knee and osteoarthritis of the hip are among the most common and probably have the greatest impact on physical function and quality of life. The one exception is OA of the spine, but it is difficult to disentangle this from all other causes of back pain which are dealt with in this chapter as a single entity. This section focuses on the burden of disease due to OA of the knee and hip.

Changes in disease occurrence

OA of the knee predominantly affects older people, usually presenting in the sixth and seventh decades. Women are affected more often than men. OA of the knee appears to be ubiquitous with little geographical variation in prevalence.[22] Projections based on the Global Burden of Disease 1990 Project suggest that OA of the knee is likely to become the fourth most important cause of disability in women and the eighth most important cause in men in developed countries in the next decade or so.[23] This is mainly as a consequence of an ageing population, but also because some of the risk factors for OA of the knee are becoming more prevalent. The main risk factors for the development of this condition (apart from increasing age and female gender) are obesity and previous knee injury.[24] There is thus scope for the primary prevention of OA of the knee and, given the projected size of the problem, this should become a major healthcare aim. Obesity is also a risk factor for progression.[24] There is evidence that weight reduction can reduce the risk of subsequent OA of the knee and also slow the progression of existing disease. However, results from targeted weight loss are generally poor and most individuals continue to gain weight. Benefits are more likely to come from societal changes (i.e. a downward shift in weight within the population). There are also opportunities to reduce the incidence of knee injury particularly within occupational settings and in sport.

OA of the hip, by contrast, shows clear geographical variation with lower rates of radiographic disease in Asian and African populations. The prevalence is approximately equal in the two sexes, and it occurs over a wide age range. Data from Malmö, Sweden suggest that the prevalence of OA of the hip has remained stable for the last 30 years.[25] Known risk factors include anatomical factors such as congenital dislocation of the hip, previous Perthe's disease, leg-length discrepancies and acetabular dysplasia. Opinions differ as to the proportion of cases of OA of the hip that can be attributed to these local causes. It is possible that some of the geographical variation in occurrence of OA of the hip can be attributed to differences in the frequency of risk factors – for example the practice of carrying babies astride the mother's back (which is common in Africa and China) may lead to development of a deeper acetabulum, and squatting may protect against hip OA. Obesity is not strongly associated with OA of the hip. There is an increased risk of OA of the hip amongst farmers. There is probably little further scope for the primary prevention of this disease.

Changes in disease course

Many cases of OA of the knee are relatively mild and do not progress.[26] However, a proportion of patients do develop severe joint destruction with associated pain and disability. It could be argued that it would be more cost effective to aim to slow the progression of OA of the knee (secondary prevention) than to try and prevent all incident cases (primary prevention). However, apart from obesity, it is likely that most risk factors for the progression of this disease are at present unknown. The natural history of OA of the hip is also very variable. It has been suggested that most OA of the hip progresses very slowly and that a minority of cases enter a rapidly progressive stage at various time points. At present the risk factors for entering the rapidly progressive phase are unknown and so the opportunities for secondary prevention are small. It seems likely that drug therapy which slows the rate of cartilage breakdown will become available during the next few years. When that happens there is likely to be a flurry of research directed at establishing what proportion of patients with large joint OA should receive these medications and at what stage in their disease.

For the time being joint replacement surgery (tertiary prevention) is the best available treatment for patients with severe OA of the knee or the hip. There is and will continue to be an increasing need for joint replacement surgery, which has major cost implications. In the UK it has been estimated that the number of total hip replacements required will increase by 40% over the next 30 years as a consequence of demographic changes alone, assuming that the present age and sex specific arthroplasty rates are maintained.[27] The requirement for knee replacements is likely to escalate even faster because there is greater evidence of unmet need at present, and the prevalence of the primary indication (OA of the knee) will increase dramatically.

There are a number of problems associated with estimating the need for major joint replacement surgery, including the current lack of evidence-based guidelines for surgery, variations and inequities in use.[28] Hip arthroplasty rates in Sweden are approximately double those in the UK.[27] There is no evidence of any differences in the frequency or severity of the underlying disease and indications for surgery are similar. The difference may therefore be due to variations in referral patterns from primary to secondary care, or to differences in the availability of operating time or surgeons. There is evidence that age, ethnicity and obesity affect surgical decisions.[29]

In conclusion, the number of people with OA worldwide is likely to rise dramatically in the next decade or so as a consequence of demographic changes. In particular the absolute and relative number of people with OA of the knee will escalate rapidly, especially if current trends in the prevalence of obesity persist. Until the advent of effective secondary preventive measures the need for major joint replacement surgery (and for orthopaedic surgeons) will rise year on year. If this need cannot be met then the burden of pain and disability due to OA within the community will mount.

Osteoporosis

Osteoporosis is, and will continue to be, one of the most prevalent musculoskeletal disorders. Bone mass reaches a peak in women towards the end of their third decade of life and is then maintained at a relatively constant level until the menopause. Immediately following the menopause bone loss begins to occur and this decline continues until the end of life. A fall in bone density also occurs in men in association with increasing age and male osteoporosis is an increasing problem.

Changes in disease occurrence

Table 2.1 shows the prevalence of osteoporosis in postmenopausal women in Rochester, Minnesota, USA. As life expectancy increases, more and more women are developing significant bone fragility which is manifest as fractures especially of the wrist, vertebra and hip. Hip fractures in the elderly are already acknowledged to be a major public health problem in the more developed countries. The majority can be attributed to osteoporosis. Cooper et al.[31] have attempted to estimate the likely numbers of hip fractures in 2025 and 2050 based on existing age and sex specific data on hip fracture rates and projections of the population structure in different regions of the world. The number of fractures is destined to increase globally but there will be a relative decrease in the proportion of the world's fractures which occur in Europe and North America and a dramatic rise in the proportion occurring in Asia (Table 2.2). These projections do not

Table 2.1 Prevalence of osteoporosis in postmenopausal women (data from Melton et al.[30])

Age (yr)	Osteoporosis at any site (%)	Osteoporosis at the hip (%)
50–59	14.8	3.9
60–69	21.6	8.0
70–79	38.5	24.5
80+	70.0	47.6

Table 2.2 Projected number of hip fractures for eight geographical regions up to 2050 (data Cooper et al.[31])

Year	Latin America	North America	Europe	Russia	Middle East	Asia	Africa	Oceania	Total
1990									
Number	96 457	358 296	407 223	152 403	52 584	572 417	7714	13 203	1 660 297
% of total	6	22	25	9	3	34	0.5	1	
2025									
Number	321 447	669 044	651 462	259 867	192 056	1 790 682	29 742	27 422	3 941 722
% of total	8	17	17	7	5	45	1	1	
2050									
Number	655 648	763 228	725 189	309 414	435 951	2 919 768	75 905	43 898	5 929 001
% of total	11	13	12	5	7	49	1	1	

take account of any secular changes in age and sex specific incidence. There is evidence that the incidence of hip fractures may have reached a plateau in Europe and North America whereas it still appears to be rising steeply in Asia.[32] Thus, the burden of hip fractures in Asia may be even greater than these projections.

Changes in disease course

The above projections do not take account of, or estimate, the likely take-up of effective measures for primary and secondary prevention of osteoporosis. Box 2.2 lists the potentially modifiable risk factors for

---

Box 2.2 Risk factors for the development of osteoporosis

May be modifiable:
- Oestrogen deficiency
- Premature menopause
- Amenorrhea
- Prolonged immobility
- Smoking
- Excess alcohol
- Dietary factors
- Low body mass index
- Susceptibility to falls
- Secondary causes, e.g. steroids

Non-modifiable:
- Age
- Ethnicity
- Genetic predisposition
- Previous fragility fracture
- Short stature

---

osteoporosis. Strategies to reduce the incidence of fragility fractures can be population based or targeted at individuals at high risk. General approaches to improve lifestyle may be targeted at the entire adult population with recommendations to increase exercise, ensure adequate calcium and vitamin D intake, stop smoking, reduce alcohol consumption and minimise external hazards both within and outside the home to reduce the risk of falls. Those at high risk of osteoporosis may be treated with hormone replacement therapy or bisphosphonates.

There are also opportunities for secondary prevention once osteoporosis has been diagnosed.

In conclusion the prevalence of osteoporosis and the incidence of hip fractures is likely to rise over the next few decades as a consequence of the increase in the world population and the changes in age structure. The brunt of these increases will fall on countries in Asia. There is evidence that the age and sex specific incidence of osteoporosis may now be stable in Europe and North America, but is continuing to rise in Asia. It is likely that the same rise is occurring in Latin America. People of African origin seem to be relatively protected against osteoporosis and this is likely to continue. There is scope for the primary prevention of osteoporosis and this needs to be considered by all regions in which the burden is otherwise likely to rise.

Back pain

Unlike RA, OA and osteoporosis, back pain is a symptom rather than a diagnosis. There are many recognised pathological causes of back pain. Nevertheless, in the individual case, it is usually impossible to ascribe the pain to a single cause. Correlations between anatomical abnormalities (for example, degenerative changes seen on x ray), and symptoms and disability are poor. It has proved more helpful to study the occurrence and prognosis of back pain as a whole than to try and disentangle the epidemiology of the separate causes of back pain. The epidemiology of back pain is intriguing. It is much more difficult to compare studies of the occurrence of back pain than it is those of RA, OA or osteoporosis because there is no standard definition of back pain. Indeed there is no standard definition of the back! In Britain and North America low back pain and neck pain are recognised as separate entities whereas in Germany all spinal pain is considered as a single entity. Nevertheless it is clear that low back pain is a ubiquitous health problem and, after the common cold, it is probably the most frequent condition to affect humankind. Up to 80% of the world's population can expect to experience an episode of back pain during their lifetimes.

Changes in disease occurrence

In most developed countries low back pain is a major cause of disability, especially in adults of working age. In Britain, during the decade to 1993, outpatient clinic attendances for back pain rose fivefold and the number of days of incapacity due to back disorders for which social security benefits were paid more than doubled.[33] A recent comparison of two similar British studies conducted 10 years apart found that the one year age standardised prevalence of self-reported back pain had risen by 12.7%.[34] The prevalence of severe back related disability in the same period was essentially unchanged. The authors favoured the explanation that cultural changes have led to a greater awareness of minor back symptoms and an increased willingness to view them as abnormal and so report them as an illness. Croft highlights the challenge for the next decade of how to understand and modify beliefs and health-seeking behaviour, while keeping faith with the person with the pain.[35]

The WHO and International League of Associations for Rheumatology (ILAR) supported Community Oriented Program for the Control of Rheumatic Disease (COPCORD) has conducted epidemiological surveys in a variety of developing countries using similar methodology. The results of these suggest that the prevalence of back pain may vary substantially from place to place (Figure 2.7). Nevertheless there is still the possibility that people in different settings may interpret the questions about pain differently, either because of nuances of translation or because the words 'ache' and 'pain' have varying meanings in different socioeconomic or cultural groups.

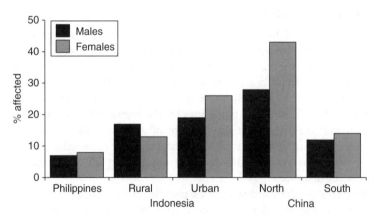

Figure 2.7 Prevalence of back pain in Asia Pacific region: COPCORD studies.

There are many risk factors associated with back pain. It has been estimated that up to 90% of people with back pain have mechanical back pain.[36] In the remaining 10% the pain can be ascribed to a systemic illness or structural abnormality such as lumbar stenosis, osteoporotic fracture or malignancy. Mechanical low back pain has been defined as pain secondary to misuse of a normal anatomical structure. Apart from structural abnormalities of the spine, and age and gender, risk factors for back pain fall into two broad categories: mechanical/occupational and psychosocial.[36] Even within the occupational category psychosocial factors play a part, with those who are dissatisfied with their jobs having a higher frequency of pain. Jobs which involve heavy lifting and those which involve working in awkward positions are also associated with a higher frequency of back pain. Psychosocial factors include depression and lower socioeconomic status. Obesity and smoking are also risk factors for back pain. This list would appear to offer opportunities for primary prevention but there is no evidence yet of a successful programme having been developed.

Back pain is predominantly a problem of the working age group. The proportion of people in this age group is destined to fall (Figure 2.6). However, with the overall increase in the world population even within this age group, and the trends outlined above in back pain prevalence, it seems likely that the burden of back pain (and of other regional and chronic pain conditions) is likely to rise.

Changes in disease course

Most episodes of back pain are self-limiting and not incapacitating. Over half of all episodes of back pain last less than one week and 90% of individuals have recovered within eight weeks. However, beyond this time recovery becomes less and less likely. Back pain that has persisted beyond 12 months is likely to be intractable. A number of developed countries have introduced guidelines for the management of acute back pain which are directed at the concept of early mobilisation and pain management using cognitive-behavioural therapy approaches. There is no evidence as yet that this has had any impact on the community burden of disease.

Regrettably, the burden of back pain is set to increase, particularly if those in the less developed countries adopt the same attitude to pain as is prevalent in the more developed countries.

Conclusions

The burden of all four conditions highlighted in this chapter is likely to increase over the next few decades. Part of the increase will be due to the absolute increase in the size of the world's population, but more is attributable to changes in the age structure of the population. Given that these changes in population structure are probably inevitable, can anything be done to reduce the predicted burden of pain and disability? Some opportunities for primary and secondary prevention have been highlighted and will be developed in subsequent chapters of this book. Population based strategies require action by governments and education of the public about the likely benefits. None of these changes, particularly changes in lifestyle, can be mandated and so "ownership" of the policies by the community is essential. It has become the fashion to set targets for health improvement prior to the introduction of programmes of primary, secondary or tertiary prevention in the hope that these will motivate all concerned.

In January 2000 the United States Department of Health and Human Services released *Healthy People 2010*, the nation's health goals for this decade.[37] The report includes 467 specific objectives in 28 "focus" areas – one of which is arthritis, osteoporosis and chronic back conditions. The WHO for Europe has decided to be more focussed and has issued 21 targets for the twenty-first century;[38] this also may be too many, and many regions have chosen to focus on only five to ten. The British Government has selected only four – cancer, coronary heart disease and stroke, accidents and mental illness. Time will tell which approach works better. Musculoskeletal disorders are omitted from the focussed British approach, but this may be of no consequence if an overambitious approach would bring no gain. Many of the changes in lifestyle advocated for the prevention of cancer and heart disease would also benefit bone and joint health. It is important not to fall into the trap of thinking that improvements in musculoskeletal health can only be achieved in the context of such political plans. It remains to be seen whether target setting actually makes any difference to health.[39]

The monitoring of targets requires the availability of data on the occurrence and outcome of the disorders in question. The Global Burden of Disease 1990 Project found that there are many parts of the world for which there are no data on musculoskeletal disorders occurrence, and this needs to be rectified. There is a particular need for information from South America and Africa. However, it is not necessary for every town to conduct its own survey, nor for every patient to be monitored intensively with multiple outcome measures. One anxiety about the enormous scope of the US plan[38] is that it will divert resources from health improvement activities to the tracking of outcomes. Much is currently known about the effective primary, secondary and tertiary prevention of musculoskeletal disorders and could be implemented within existing resources. Additional resources are needed and a proportion should be directed at the acquisition of further data, but the majority should be directed at alleviating and preventing the problem itself.

References

1 World Bank. *World development report 1993; investing in health.* New York: Oxford University Press, 1993.
2 Murray CJL, Lopez AD, eds. *Global comparative assessments in the health sector.* Geneva: World Health Organization, 1994.
3 World Health Organization. *International Classification of Diseases Version 9.* Geneva: WHO, 1979.
4 United Nations Population Division, Department of Economic and Social Affairs. *World population prospects. The 1998 Revision.* New York: United Nations.
5 Symmons DPM, Harrison BJ. Risk factors for the development of inflammatory polyarthritis and rheumatoid arthritis. *Rheumatology* 2000;**39**:835–43.
6 Silman A. Primary prevention of rheumatoid arthritis. In: Wrigley RD, ed. *The primary prevention of rheumatic diseases.* Carnforth: Parthenon Publishing, 1994;229–40.
7 Beasley RP, Bennett PH, Chin Lin C. Low prevalence of rheumatoid arthritis in Chinese. Prevalence survey in a rural community. *J Rheumatol* 1983;(suppl. 10):11–15.
8 Ollier W, Thomson W. Population genetics of rheumatoid arthritis. *Rheum Dis Clin North Am* 1992;**18**:741–9.
9 Solomon L, Robin G, Valkenburg HA. Rheumatoid arthritis in an urban South African Negro population. *Ann Rheum Dis* 1975;**34**:128–35.
10 Lau E, Symmons D, Bankhead C, MacGregor A, Donnan S, Silman A. Low prevalence of rheumatoid arthritis in the urbanised Chinese people of Hong Kong. *J Rheumatol* 1993;**20**:1133–7.
11 Silman AJ. Has the incidence of rheumatoid arthritis fallen in the United Kingdom? *Br J Rheumatol* 1988;**27**:77–8.
12 Dugowson CE, Koepsall TD, Voigt LF, Bley L, Nelson JL, Daling JR. Rheumatoid arthritis in women: incidence rates in a group health co-operative, Seattle, Washington 1987–9. *Arthritis Rheum* 1991;**34**:1502–7.
13 Spector TD, Hochberg M. The protective effect of the oral contraceptive pill on rheumatoid arthritis: an overview of the analytic epidemiological studies using meta-analysis. *J Clin Epidemiol* 1990;**43**:1221–30.
14 Kaipiainen-Seppänen O, Aho K, Isomäki H, Laakso M. Shift in the incidence of rheumatoid arthritis toward elderly patients in Finland during 1975–90. *Clin Exp Rheumatol* 1996;**14**:537–42.
15 Symmons DPM, Barrett EM, Bankhead CR, Scott DGI, Silman AJ. The incidence of rheumatoid arthritis in the United Kingdom: results from the Norfolk Arthritis Register. *Br J Rheumatol* 1994;**33**:735–9.

16 Egsmose C, Lund B, Borg G et al. Patients with rheumatoid arthritis benefit from early second-line therapy: 5 year follow-up of a prospective double blind placebo controlled study. *J Rheumatol* 1995;**22**:2208–13.

17 Lindqvist E, Eberhardt K. Mortality in rheumatoid arthritis patients with disease onset in the 1980s. *Ann Rheum Dis* 1999;**58**:11–14.

18 Wallberg-Jonsson S, Ohman ML, Dahlqvist SR. Cardiovascular morbidity and mortality in patients with sero-positive rheumatoid arthritis in Northern Sweden. *J Rheumatol* 1997;**24**:445–51.

19 Tugwell P, Wells G, Strand V et al. Clinical improvement as reflected in measures of function and health-related quality of life following treatment with leflunomide compared with methotrexate in patients with rheumatoid arthritis. *Arthritis Rheum* 2000;**43**:506–14.

20 Elliott MJ, Maini RN, Feldmann M et al. Randomised double-blind comparison of chimeric monoclonal antibody to tumour necrosis factor alpha (cA2) versus placebo in rheumatoid arthritis. *Lancet* 1994;**344**: 1105–10.

21 Moreland LW, Schiff MH, Baumgartner SW et al. Etanercept therapy in rheumatoid arthritis: a randomised controlled trial. *Ann Intern Med* 1999;**130**:478–86.

22 McCarney R, Croft P. Knee pain. In: Crombie IK, Croft PR, Linton SJ, LeResche L, von Korff M, eds. *Epidemiology of Pain*. Seattle: IASP, 1999.

23 Murray CJL, Lopez A. *The global burden of disease*. Geneva: World Health Organization, 1997.

24 Cooper C, Snow S, McAlindon T et al. Risk factors for the incidence and progression of radiographic knee osteoarthritis. *Arthritis Rheum* 2000;**43**:995–1000.

25 Danielson LG, Lindberg HL. Prevalence of coxarthrosis in an urban population during four decades. *Clin Orthop* 1997;**342**:106–10.

26 Felson D. The course of osteoarthritis and the factors that affect it. *Rheum Dis Clin North Am* 1993;**19**:607–15.

27 Birrell F, Johnell O, Silman A. Projecting the need for hip replacement over the next three decades: influence of changing demography and threshold for surgery. *Ann Rheum Dis* 1999;**58**:569–72.

28 Dieppe P, Basler HD, Chard J et al. Knee replacement surgery for osteoarthritis: effectiveness, practice variations, indications and possible determinants of utilisation. *Rheumatology* 1999;**38**:73–83.

29 Wilson MG, May DS, Kelly JJ. Racial differences in the use of total knee arthroplasty for osteoarthritis amongst older Americans. *Ethnic Dis* 1994;**4**:57–67.

30 Melton LJ III, Chrischilles EA, Cooper C, Lane AW, Riggs BL. How many women have osteoporosis? *J Bone Miner Res* 1992;**7**:1005–10.

31 Cooper C, Campion G, Melton LJ III. Hip fractures in the elderly: a world-wide projection. *Osteoporosis Int* 1992;**2**:285–9.

32 Lau EMC, Cooper C, Fund H, Lam D, Tsang KK. Hip fracture in Hong Kong over the last decade – a comparison with the UK. *J Publ Health Med* 1999;**21**:249–50.

33 Clinical Standards Advisory Group. *Epidemiology review: the epidemiology and cost of back pain*. London: HMSO, 1994.

34 Palmer KT, Walsh K, Bendall H, Cooper C, Coggon D. Back pain in Britain: comparison of two prevalence surveys at an interval of 10 years. *Br Med J* 2000;**320**:1577–8.

35 Croft P. Is life becoming more of a pain? *Br Med J* 2000;**320**:1552–3.

36 Borenstein DG. Low back pain. In: Klippel JH, Dieppe PA, eds. *Rheumatology*, 2nd ed. London: Mosby International, 1998: Section 4.3.

37 US Department of Health and Human Services. *Healthy People 2010*. Washington DC: US Department of Health and Human Services.

38 World Health Organization Europe. *Health 21 – health for all in the 21st century*. Copenhagen: WHO Regional Office for Europe, 1999.

39 McKee M, Fulop N. On target for health? *Br Med J* 2000;**320**:327–8.

3: From basic science to the future bedside: the potential of developments in bioscience and technology

FERDINAND C BREEDVELD

Physicians who have recently changed their armamentarium for the treatment of musculoskeletal diseases will have to continue to do so. The rapid developments in molecular biology and computer assisted chemistry allow the design of therapies targeted at molecules that play an essential role in arthritis and related conditions. Targeted therapies follow the most recent appreciation of diseases, which is a dynamic situation given the fast growing insight in the nature of these diseases. The best chance of finding a therapy that cures is to completely understand the cause of a disease. However, despite intensive research this has only been achieved to a certain extent in diseases such as gout and infectious arthritides. In other diseases such as rheumatoid arthritis, osteoarthritis, bone loss and chronic pain syndromes it seems that the more we know the more we realise the complexity of these diseases. The best chance of achieving complete understanding of a disease will come from creative interactions between molecular biological and epidemiological lines of research. This does not imply that before complete insight has been achieved no therapeutic breakthroughs can be obtained. Bone and joint diseases are known to be mediated by a vast array of soluble factors and cells that act to recruit more cells at the site of destruction or inflammation. The signals used by the cells are known and selective blockage has already established great improvements in the treatment of arthritis and bone loss. These achievements have opened the way for more refined targeted therapies. Extracellular signals are transduced intracellularly by various pathways resulting in alterations in transcription factors that bind to genes to induce expression and subsequently cellular effector functions. Therapies targeted at any of these steps both upstream and downstream of the mediators of destruction and inflammation will prove to be of benefit in the near future. Such pharmaceutical therapies may be delivered simply by the oral administration of small molecules, parenteral administration of large proteins or organ specific drug production via gene therapy.

Chronic arthritis is generally regarded as an autoimmune disease. These diseases exhibit defined immunological reactions against self tissues as a major component of their pathogenesis. The holy grail of therapy for clinical immunologists is a targeted treatment that would destroy those parts of the immune system that cause harm and leave alone that part that protects the body against infection and cancer. That ideal may be realised by therapies using immune ablation and therapies using haematopoietic stem cells.

This chapter will provide a summary of the lines of research in bioscience and technology that underlie the targeted therapies of the future.

Genetic research in bone and joint diseases

Diseases such as rheumatoid arthritis, osteoarthritis or osteoporosis have a complex pathophysiological background. In these diseases there is no single set of conditions sufficient to induce disease. The primary goal of researchers is to find successful interventions that may prevent or cure disease. Such successful interventions may affect all factors in the pathogenesis which themselves are not generally considered as causes of disease. An example is blockage of tumour necrosis factor (TNF), a cytokine needed for host defence, which proved to be a successful therapy for rheumatoid arthritis.[1,2] The second goal is to be able to predict the effect of targeted interventions in disease mechanisms. Here the objective is to describe the hierarchy of participating mechanisms that predict the performance of the system. Finally all the participants in the pathogenetic system should be described. It is now realised that genetic studies are helpful in defining the essential conditions underlying the diseases of bones and joints. Familial clustering is one of the primary observations which suggested that genetic variants influence disease susceptibility. Genetic studies, for example association studies with genetic markers or segregation studies of genetic markers and disease within families, can help to identify the involved genes. These studies will identify the polymorphic genes that are associated with the disease and these will be the critical elements on which hypotheses on hierarchy within disease mechanisms will be based.

During the last decade we have witnessed important breakthroughs in genetic research. The completion of the human genome project demonstrates that 30 000 different genes are present and have yielded information on the relative location of most genes to each other.[3,4] Information on all the variants within these genes is rapidly growing, and it is expected that the loci responsible for these diseases will be identified in the next decade. However, the understanding of the precise role of these factors in the pathophysiology of diseases will take considerably more time. It can be expected that clinical experimentalists will directly use the information coming out of these lines of research for the design of targeted therapeutic interventions.

Emerging therapeutic targets

Extracellular signals

Of the many cytokines thought to contribute to the inflammatory or degenerative changes that occur in the diseases of the motion apparatus, TNF has emerged as being of major pathological significance.[5] For example, TNF was found to be overproduced at the site of rheumatoid inflammation and many lines of preclinical research were consistent with a pathogenetic role. In particular, TNF promotes the resorption of cartilage and regulates the production of other proinflammatory mediators. A further piece of evidence that helped to illustrate the pathological role of this cytokine in arthritis was the observation that TNF transgenic mice that express human TNF in a transgenic fashion spontaneously develop arthritis that can be prevented by anti-human TNF monoclonal antibodies.[6] Confirmation of the central role of TNF in arthritis came from clinical trials with TNF antagonists. The trials showed that TNF blockage directly ameliorates clinical symptoms. Long term treatment prevents radiographic disease progression and loss of mobility.[7]

Interleukin (IL) 1 is another master cytokine in chronic destructive arthritis. Experimental work provided evidence for the conclusion that TNF and IL-1 act in series, with TNF inducing the expression of IL-1.[5] However, TNF independent IL-1 production has also been reported.[8] The relevance of this is underlined by the efficacy of anti-IL-1 treatment in preventing experimental joint destruction and total lack of chronic, erosive arthritis in IL-1 deficient mice. The attractiveness of IL-1 as a therapeutic target was finally proven by clinical trials that showed anti-inflammatory and joint protective effects of the IL-1 inhibitor IL-1 receptor antagonist.[9]

The clinical trials with TNF and IL-1 antagonists showed an unprecedented clinical efficacy in a therapy refractory patient population but the efficacy was never complete. Studies on synovial biopsies showed heterogeneous patterns of cytokine production in individual patients.[10] This argues for the existence of different disease pathways between patients. Therefore future treatment with antagonists of both IL-1 and TNF seems to be attractive. The role of other cytokines cannot be disregarded. Of interest at present are IL-17, a T cell derived cytokine that shares many properties of IL-1,[11] osteoprotegerin ligand that is a pivotal mediator of osteoclast differentiation[12] and activations, as well as IL-18 that is being produced by stromal cells and sustains a T_1 helper cell (TH1) response that is so characteristic for the rheumatoid inflammation.[13] It is tempting to speculate that tailormade cytokine directed treatment will be applicable in the future. Other forms of combination therapy such as those targeted at TNF and at the pathogenic T cell response may be attractive as well.

Intracellular signals

One of the most important inducers of inflammation is the transcription factor nuclear factor κB (NF-κB). NF-κB is involved in the expression of proinflammatory cytokines, enzymes and adhesions molecules.[14] Moreover, NF-κB can prevent apoptosis and has therefore been implicated in synovial hyperplasia.[15] In the rheumatoid synovium NF-κB is found predominantly in the nuclei of synovial macrophages, both in the synovial lining, the sublining and in endothelial cells. The location in the nucleus indicates that activation has taken place. NF-κB also plays a key role in the periarticular bone erosions for rheumatoid arthritis. Binding of RANKL (receptor activator of NF-κB ligand) to its cognate receptor, RANK, also leads to activation of NF-κB. Many lines of research are followed to discover specific inhibitors of NF-κB. This may be achieved by inhibiting essential signalling pathways for its activation, or by blocking its translocation to the nucleus or competitive inhibition with decoy oligonucleotides. Promising results have been obtained from animal models in which inhibition of NF-κB by decoys or by an IκB (inhibitor of κB) repressor successfully reduced the expression of experimentally induced arthritis in rats.[15] Interest here is further stimulated by the observation that several established antirheumatic drugs influence NF-κB activation. Glucocorticosteroids increase IκB expression and retain NF-κB in the cytoplasm thereby inhibiting the expression of proinflammatory genes. Sulfasalazine and leflunomide also interfere with the NF-κB signalling pathway by inhibiting IκB degradation or by preventing nuclear translocation of NF-κB.[16,17]

TNF is produced as a transmembrane protein which is cleaved from the membrane by the metalloprotease TNF converting enzyme (TACE) to form a soluble TNF molecule.[18] By crosslinking three surface receptors TNF induces various effector functions that are relevant for amplifying the rheumatoid inflammation. Following crosslinking of TNF receptors, signalling proteins are recruited, the TNF receptor associated factors (TRAF) that in the end activate the transcription factors NF-κB and activate protein 1 (AP-1).[19] In addition to molecules within the pathway of NF-κB activation, TRAF proteins are potential therapeutic targets within the TNF receptor signal transduction pathway. TRAF blockage could be more specific than the blockage of TNF itself by blocking only specific TRAFs in cells active in rheumatoid arthritis without altering TNF signals needed in the defenses against microorganisms.

Mitogen activated protein kinase (MAPK) pathways include the extracellular signal regulated kinases (ERKs), the c-Jun amino-terminal kinases (JNKs) and p38 MAPK.[20] These kinases are key signalling enzymes that the cells use to adapt rapidly to inflammatory and stressful conditions. In rheumatoid arthritis p38 kinase is involved in AP-1 activation that leads to collagenase gene expression. Molecules aimed at inhibiting AP-1 are presently under development. Rheumatoid synovial tissue and synoviocytes of patients with rheumatoid arthritis and osteoarthritis stimulated with IL-1 show phosphorylated p38 MAPK, JNK and ERKs. TNF also induces phosphorylation.

A group of orally available pyridinyl imidazol compounds specifically inhibit p38 MAPK.[21] These drugs function by competitive binding to the ATP pocket of both active and inactive forms of the kinase. Inhibitors of p38 MAP kinase can reduce production of the proinflammatory cytokines TNF, IL-1, IL-6 and IL-8 from stimulated peripheral blood mononuclear cells and rheumatoid synovial fibroblasts.[22] Prophylactic or therapeutic administration of these compounds was effective in reducing the severity of induced animal models of arthritis. Several of these compounds are now in clinical development.

Metalloproteinases

Cartilage and bone destruction in rheumatoid arthritis and osteoarthritis is considered to be mediated by overproduction of metalloproteinases (MMPs). MMPs include more than 25 enzymes grouped as gelatinases, stromalysines and collagenases that are released as inactive molecules which become active when the propeptide is cleaved.[23] They play a key role in normal connective tissue remodelling and are therefore usually under tight regulation with respect to release, activation and inhibition by their natural inhibitors – alpha$_2$ macroglobulin and the tissue inhibitors of metalloproteinases (TIMPs). One of the first questions in developing a MMP inhibitor is determining the in vivo relevance of specific MMPs in a specific disease.[24] Three collagenases (MMP-1, MMP-8 and MMP-13) have been identified in human cartilage and their levels have been shown to be increased in osteoarthritis. All collagenases are active on collagen fibrils but their biochemical activity and distribution in arthritic cartilage differs in a way that it has been suggested that MMP-1 is primarily involved in destruction and MMP-13 in tissue remodelling.[25] Development of MMP inhibitors has been based on known interactions between the enzyme and their substrates/inhibitors in order to design molecules that specifically block the active site. In this design choices have to be made in the intensity and the specificity of the inhibition.

For many of the MMP inhibitors developed for a number of indications, the therapeutic efficacy in animal models of induced disease has been impressive. However, the application of the early inhibitors was limited by the relatively poor bioavailability, immunogenicity and toxicity. The characterisation of orally available broad range MMP inhibitors such as marimastat and Trocade has proved important data.[26,27] Some other agents have also shown to inhibit MMP production. Bisphosphonates inhibit MMP-2. Minocycline and doxycycline appear to be active against collagenase and gelatinases. The effect of these compounds on MMP inhibition is not yet fully exploited.

Inhibition of TACE and therefore blocking of the processing of the precursor to the active soluble form of TNF results in the elimination of soluble TNF and achieves the same or greater efficacy in an animal model of inflammation as that seen with the available TNF antagonists.[28] From the standpoint of ease of administration and reduced costs of therapy, an orally administered selective small inhibitor of TNF would be desirable. A series of orally available potent TACE inhibitors are currently in clinical development.

The ongoing clinical trials with enzyme inhibitors will provide a better understanding of key issues in these arthritic diseases. The trials should provide answers about whether one or a spectrum of MMPs should be inhibited or whether blockage of other disease mechanisms upstream of MMP production is more effective.

Other targets

Many pathogenetic mechanisms involving cells and mediators of inflammation and destruction are involved in arthritis. Targeting any of them may reveal an interesting therapeutic possibility. An example is interference with angiogenesis. One of the earliest characteristics of early inflammation in destructive arthritis is the formation of new vessels. It has been envisioned that direct vascular targeting may become a reality.[29] It is also possible that efforts aimed at down-regulating the cytokines that regulate vessel formation offer a novel therapy. A second example is inhibition of chemokines. These molecules produced by inflammatory cells attract more inflammatory cells towards the site of inflammation. Several inhibitors of chemokines are already in clinical development.[30] The best example concerns T cell targeted therapy. Particularly in the case of inflammatory rheumatic conditions T cells are considered to play a central role in driving inflammation. Most trials that aimed at the depletion of these cells from the joint have proven to be unsuccessful. Evidence accumulated that anti-T cell antibodies need to be administered at sufficient dose, frequency and duration to achieve clinical improvement.[31] Well designed trials may be expected to result in clinical improvement. Alternative T cell directed therapies target the signals needed by T cells to become activated. Blockage of the T cell costimulation makes the cell permanently unresponsive. CTLA4Ig is a molecule that blocks the T cell stimulation for the essential interaction of CD28 with CD80 and was very effective in a variety of rodent models of inflammatory autoimmune diseases. Its therapeutic efficacy in patients with rheumatoid arthritis is being evaluated at present. Other T cell targeted therapies try to achieve specific tolerance of the immune system for joint tissue. Vaccination with particular antigens may induce new populations of T cells that regain this tolerance. The relevance of this approach has been demonstrated in animal models of arthritis such as the collagen induced arthritis model. Clinical trials that follow this principle are being prepared or are under way.

Gene therapy

Gene therapy can be defined as transfer of new genetic material to the cell of an individual with resulting therapeutic benefit to the individual. This therapy makes use of vectors (viruses), which enable the cellular uptake of genetic material in such a way that the genetic information can be expressed. The amount of the intended product formed by the cell is regulated by the promotor used in the vector. Promotors are regions of DNA, usually situated adjacent to the genes they regulate, that are essential for appropriate transcription. For joint diseases one could think of local or systemic gene therapy. Systemic gene therapy in which genes are transferred to extra-articular locations aims at modulation of the disease in all joints at once. Because rheumatoid arthritis is not a monogenetic defect systemic gene transfer will focus on immunomodulation rather than on strategies aimed at gene repair. When all the technical issues are addressed systemic gene therapy may be an attractive alternative for the parenteral administration of larger proteins. However, at present it is still difficult to obtain long term gene expression and to regulate the expression of genes. Local gene therapy seeks to transfer genes to tissues within the individual affected joints. A major advantage of local delivery is created by the anatomy of the joint, in which the synovial cavity borders only to cartilage and synovium. Here primarily synoviocytes are available for infections with the vectors. Localising the gene in the synovium ensures maximum therapeutic effect within the joint, making it possible to deliver safely and effectively certain proteins that may be toxic upon systemic injection. In animal models of arthritis local expression of biological response modifiers such as anti-TNF soluble FAS ligand, IL-1 receptor antagonist and IL-10 have shown to reduce inflammation in the synovium and to inhibit destruction of cartilage.[32–34] Local strategy is not hampered by the need for stable long term gene expression. When synoviocytes are brought to genetic modifications that need short expression times, such as genes that encode toxic proteins, effective local therapies can be designed with synovectomy or tissues engineering as a result. Such trials are underway.

Tissue engineering

Even in the presence of effective antirheumatic therapies in 2010, there will be patients who have developed joint damage. Therefore apart from the prevention of joint damage other strategies should be explored to rebuild the joint. Connective tissue stem cells can be brought in for differentiation towards cartilage cells hereby allowing the possibility of healing cartilage defects.[35,36] Currently the factors involved in such differentiation are being discovered. These factors can be introduced in the joint or can be applied for ex vivo differentiation of cells that are subsequently injected into the joint. The clinical efficacy of cartilage repair via injection of new cartilage cells is being explored at present. The foreseen possibility of rebuilding a joint will dramatically influence clinical decision making. Because life expectation will continue to increase, the number of patients in need of joint replacement will also increase. This will pose an interesting dilemma where a large population has to choose either joint replacement or strategies that are aimed at rebuilding a joint.

Immune ablation and haematopoietic stem cells

Intense immunosuppression (immune ablation) followed by infusion of haematopoietic stem cells is a relatively new therapeutic approach. Immune ablation has produced encouraging results in patients who have undergone transplantations because of coincidental malignancies. A great deal of prior research has already produced impressive results using transplant-based procedures in experimental animals, and suggestions to carry these encouraging results into the clinic soon followed. The hypothesis here is that a stable cure for autoimmune rheumatic diseases can be expected if the patient's autoreactive immunocompetent cells are replaced by healthy non-autoreactive cells, e.g. reprogramming the immune system.[37] The healthy new immune system must also remain unsusceptible to whatever phenomenon initially induced the immunological attack against the body. Two strategies can be followed: the intense immunosuppression followed by infusion of either the patient's own stem cells (autologous) or donor stem cells (allogeneic). Theoretically allogeneic transplantation is the most promising. Preliminary clinical observations have shown long term remissions and possible cures. However, the mortality and morbidity associated with this procedure, although decreasing steadily in other fields of medicine, are still unacceptably high for most autoimmune diseases. Autologous transplantation is now seen by many physicians as a possible therapy for severe refractory autoimmune disease because of a lower transplant related mortality and a greater feasibility. In the European Bone Marrow Transplant registry the overall survival is over 90%. Selection of patients with a less severe disease would certainly improve this but it must be considered that the procedure is designed for refractory patients who often have accumulated diffuse visceral damage. Extensive reviews have now been published on preliminary clinical experience in this therapeutic approach in rheumatoid arthritis, systemic lupus erythematosus and systemic sclerosis.[38-40] Many of the patients who were refractory to previous therapies responded favourably but remissions rather than cures were mostly obtained.[41] Further controlled clinical trials exploring the many technical variants of these therapies are clearly indicated.

Conclusions

Musculoskeletal conditions are the most common cause of severe long term pain and physical disability affecting large numbers of individuals. The goal for rheumatology in the twenty-first century is to advance the understanding of these diseases and to improve prevention and treatment. Solid research has already provided substantial advances in diagnosis and treatment, and biologically oriented research molecular markers of disease have been explored that help to diagnose diseases and to monitor disease progression and important pathophysiological pathways. Based on this insight new treatment modalities have already been investigated and proved to be effective. Many new products of the biotechnology industry deserve to be investigated in the near future. Such agents have been primarily studied in inflammatory conditions but will also be of significance in conditions such as osteoarthritis. Other developments that can be expected are the establishment of gene therapy, tissue engineering and reconstruction of the immune system by means of immune ablation and haematopoietic stem cells. The main goal is the delivery of the appropriate treatment to individual patients from the many that will be available.

References

1 Elliott MJ, Maini RN, Feldmann M *et al.* Treatment with a chimaeric monoclonal antibody to tumour necrosis factor α suppresses disease

activity in rheumatoid arthritis: results of a multi-centre, randomised, double-blind trial. *Lancet* 1994;**34**:334–42.

2 Moreland LW, Baumgartner SW, Schiff MH *et al.* Treatment of rheumatoid arthritis with a recombinant human tumor necrosis factor receptor (p75)-Fc fusion protein. *N Engl J Med* 1997;**337**:141–7.

3 International Human Genome Sequencing Consortium 2001. Initial Sequencing analysis of the human genome. *Nature* 2001;**409**:860–921.

4 Venter JC, Adams MD, Myers EW *et al.* The sequence of the human genome. *Science* 2001;**291**:1304–51.

5 Williams RO, Feldmann M, Maini RN. Cartilage destruction and bone erosion in arthritis: the role of tumour necrosis factor α. *Ann Rheum Dis* 2000;**59**(suppl. I):75–80.

6 Keffer J, Probert L, Cazlaris H *et al.* Transgenic mice expressing human tumour necrosis factor: a predictive genetic model of arthritis. *EMBO J* 1991;**10**:4025–31.

7 Lipsky PE, van der Heijde DM, St Clair EW *et al.* Infliximab and methotrexate in the treatment of rheumatoid arthritis. *N Engl J Med* 2000;**343**:1594–1602.

8 Berg van den WB. Arguments for interleukin 1 as a target in chronic arthritis. *Ann Rheum Dis* 2000;**59**(suppl. I):81–4.

9 Bresnihan B, Alvaro-Gracia JM, Cobby M *et al.* Treatment of rheumatoid arthritis with recombinant human interleukin-1 receptor antagonist. *Arthritis Rheum* 1998;**41**:2196–204.

10 Kirkham B, Portek I, Lee CS *et al.* Intraarticular variability of synovial membrane histology, immunohistology, and cytokine mRNA expression in patients with rheumatoid arthritis. *J Rheumatol* 1999;**25**:777–84.

11 Lubberts E, Joosten LAB, Chabaud M *et al.* IL-4 gene therapy for collagen arthritis suppresses synovial IL-17 and osteoprotegerin ligand and prevents bone erosion. *J Clin Invest* 2000;**105**:1697–710.

12 Gravallese EM, Goldring SR. Cellular mechanisms and the role of cytokines in bone erosions in rheumatoid arthritis. *Arthritis Rheum* 2000;**43**:2132–51.

13 Dinarello CA. Targeting interleukin 18 with interleukin 18 binding protein. *Ann Rheum Dis* 2000;**59**(suppl. I):17–20.

14 Baldwin ASJ. The transcription factor NF-κB and human disease. *J Clin Invest* 2001;**107**:3–6.

15 Miagkov AV, Kovalenko DV, Brown CE *et al.* NF-κB activation provides the potential link between inflammation and hyperplasia in the arthritic joint. *Proc Natl Acad Sci USA* 1998;**95**:13859–64.

16 Weber C, Liptay S, Wirth T *et al.* Suppression of NF-kappa B activity by sulfasalazine is mediated by direct inhibition of IkappaB kinases alpha and beta. *Gastroenterology* 2000;**119**:1209–18.

17 Manna S, Mukhopadhyay A, Aggarwal B. Leflunomide suppresses TNF-induced cellular responses: effects on NF-κB, activator protein-1, c-*Jun* N-terminal protein kinase, and apoptosis. *J Immunol* 2000; **165**:5962–9.

18 Black RA, Rauch CT, Kozlosky CJ *et al.* A metalloproteinase disintegrin that releases tumour-necrosis factor-α from cells. *Nature* 1997; **385**:729–33.

19 Inoue J, Ishida T, Tsukamoto N *et al.* Tumor necrosis factor receptor-associated factor (TRAF) family: adapter proteins that mediate cytokine signaling. *Exp Cell Res* 2000;**254**:14–24.

20 Kyriakis JM, Avruch J. Sounding the alarm: protein kinase cascades activated by stress and inflammation. *J Biol Chem* 1996;**271**:24313–16.

21 Herlaar E, Brown Z. p38 MAPK signalling cascades in inflammatory disease. *Molec Med Today* 1999;**5**:439–47.

22 Suzuki M, Tetsuka T, Yoshida S *et al.* The role of p38 mitogen-activated protein kinase in IL-6 and IL-8 production from the TNF-alpha- or IL-1 beta-stimulated rheumatoid synovial fibroblasts. *FEBS Lett* 2000;**465**:23–7.

23 Barrett AJ. Classification of peptidases. *Methods Enzymol* 1994;**244**:1–15.

24 Martel-Pelletier J, Pelletier JP. Wanted – the collagenase responsible for the destruction of the collagen network in human cartilage. *Br J Rheumatol* 1996;**35**:818–20.

25 Fernandes JC, Martel-Pelletier J, Lascau-Coman V *et al.* Collagenase-1 and collagenase-3 synthesis in normal and early experimental osteoarthritic canine cartilage: an immunohistochemical study. *J Rheumatol* 1998;**25**: 1585–94.

26 Hemmings FJ, Farhan M, Rowland J *et al.* Tolerability and pharmacokinetics of the collagenase-selective inhibitor Trocade™143 in patients with rheumatoid arthritis. *Rheumatology* 2001;**40**:537–43.

27 Denis LJ, Verweij J. Matrix metalloproteinase inhibitors: present achievements and future prospects. *Invest New Drugs* 1997;**15**:175–185.

28 Solomon KA, Covington MB, Decicco CP *et al.* The fate of pro-TNF-α following inhibition of metalloprotease dependent processing to soluble TNF-α in human monocytes. *J Immunol* 1997;**159**:4524–31.

29 Koch AE. The role of angiogenesis in rheumatoid arthritis: recent developments. *Ann Rheum Dis* 2000;**59**(suppl. I):65–71.

30 Kunkel SL, Lukacs N, Kasama T *et al.* The role of chemokines in inflammatory joint diseases. *J Leukoc Biol* 1996;**59**:6–12.

31 Kalden JR, Breedveld FC, Burkhardt H *et al.* Immunological treatment of autoimmune diseases. *Adv Immunol* 1998;**68**:333–418.

32 Ghivizzanni SC, Kang R, Hatton C *et al. In vivo* delivery of genes encoding soluble receptors for IL-1 and TNF-α results in a synergistic therapeutic effect in antigen-induced arthritis in rabbit knee. *Arthritis Rheum* 1996;**39**:S308.

33 Bandara G, Mueller GM, Galea-Lauri J *et al.* Intraarticular expression of biologically active IL-1 receptor antagonist protein by *ex vivo* gene transfer. *Proc Natl Acad Sci USA* 1993;**90**:10764–8.

34 Whalen JD, Lechman EL, Carlos CA *et al.* Adenoviral transfer of the viral IL-10 gene periarticularly to mouse paws suppresses development of CIA in both injected and uninjected paws. *J Immunol* 1999;**162**:3625–32.

35 Hunziker EB. Articular cartilage repair, are the intrinsic biological constraints undermining this process unsuperable? *Osteoarthr Cartilage* 1999;**7**:15–28.

36 Pittenger MF, Mackay AM, Beck SC *et al.* Multilineage potential of mesenchymal stem cells. *Science* 1999;**284**:143–7.

37 Marmont AM. Immunoablation followed or not by hematopoietic stem cells as an intense therapy for severe autoimmune diseases. New perspectives, new problems. *Haematologica* 2001;**86**:337–45.
38 Bekkum van DW. Short analytical review. New opportunities for treatment of severe autoimmune diseases: bone marrow transplantation. *Clin Immunol Immunopathol* 1998;**89**:1–10.
39 Tyndall A, Milliken S. Bone marrow transplantation for rheumatoid arthritis. *Established Rheumatoid Arthritis*, 1999;**13**:719–35.
40 Tyndall A, Gratwohl A. Blood and marrow stem cell transplantation in autoimmune diseases: a consensus report written on behalf of European League against Rheumatism (EULAR) and the European Group for Blood and Marrow Transplantation. *Bone Marrow Transplant* 1997; **19**:643–5.
41 Verburg RJ, Kruize AA, van den Hoogen FJ *et al*. High-dose chemotherapy and autologous hematopoietic stem cell transplantation in patients with rheumatoid arthritis. *Arthritis Rheum* 2001;**44**:754–60.

4: The future diagnosis and management of rheumatoid arthritis

PIET LCM van RIEL

Rheumatoid arthritis (RA) is a chronic systemic inflammatory disease of unknown origin with a highly variable presentation. Its main manifestation is a synovitis of the peripheral joints. The disease usually starts in the small joints of the hands and feet, and gradually all the other, larger joints may get involved as well. This causes for the patient not only a lot of complaints such as pain and stiffness but it has also a huge impact on mobility and psychosocial well being. Next to these articular features, frequently extra-articular features such as subcutaneous nodules, vasculitis, neurological impairment and internal organ involvement are present. Sometimes this extra-articular involvement may dominate and overshadow the joint manifestations of the disease. This means that in addition to the joint complaints the patients may suffer from constitutional complaints such as fatigue, weight loss and fever, and/or features relating to organ involvement like dyspnoea, dry eyes and hepatic failure. The inflammatory process is in principle reversible, however if it is not possible to suppress the disease activity completely soon after the start of the disease than the joints will be irreversibly damaged. Depending on the extent of the damage and the kind of joints involved this will cause additional functional restrictions. The consequence of this is that even if a complete cure of the disease becomes possible in the future, this means that all those patients with RA who already have destructive changes of their joints will only partially benefit from this.

As the cause of RA is still not known and no cure exists at present, this directs the management of this disease. In most cases the treatment is multidisciplinary, as apart from the rheumatologist a vast number of medical and allied health professionals are also involved (Box 4.1).

> **Box 4.1** Members of the multidisciplinary team
> - Rheumatologist
> - Nurse
> - Occupational therapist
> - Physical therapist
> - Social worker
> - Psychologist/psychiatrist
> - Neurologist
> - Orthopaedic surgeon
> - General physician
> - Podiatrist

In conclusion there are still many uncertainties in the diagnosis and management of RA, which gives scope for a huge number of challenges. As a result, hopefully this may lead to improvements in the management of patients with RA.

Pathogenesis

RA arthritis has a complex aetiology in which different factors interact. The current working hypothesis is that persons with a certain genetic susceptibility do develop RA when they encounter one or more appropriate environmental triggers.[1] Earlier studies from families with RA and twins have shown that genetic factors play a role in the pathogenesis of RA.[2] Studies from different populations have shown that a number of HLA-DRB1 alleles are associated with RA. Subsequent studies have made clear that all these alleles had in common a highly conserved sequence of amino acids in the third hypervariable region of their DRB1 chain – this is referred to as the shared epitope (SE) hypothesis.[3]

It is not sure whether the genetic factors that may code for susceptibility to RA are different from those that influence the subsequent disease course (see "Prognostic criteria" below). In some community based studies no association could be found between HLA-DR4 and RA, while an association in those populations was found with the severity of the disease.[4,5]

The rapid development of techniques in the field of molecular biology has made it possible to screen the human genome for alleles which may be associated with RA. Hopefully this will lead to the identification of additional susceptibility genes which may give us further clues to help us elucidate the pathogenesis of RA.

Management

The management of RA has been changed dramatically in past decades and will do so further in the near future. Within the management of the disease the following items need to be distinguished: diagnosis of the disease, prognostic factors, therapeutic interventions and disease course monitoring.

Diagnosis

As the cause of RA is not known the diagnosis is made by applying American College of Rheumatology classification criteria.[6] The diagnosis RA can be made if the patient fulfils at least four out of the seven criteria. Rheumatoid arthritis can therefore better be seen as a syndrome rather than a disease; in other words RA is a repository of inflammatory joint diseases due to many different causes. In the past several diseases which have been called RA were identified as a separate disease due to carefully studying the clinical presentation of the disease and performing epidemiological studies. Examples of such diseases are rubella arthritis and Lyme disease.[7,8]

As many studies have shown that therapeutic interventions early in the disease course lead to earlier disease control and therefore less joint damage, it is important to make the diagnosis of RA in a patient with joint symptoms as soon as possible. The classification criteria have been used for this purpose although they are not designed for it as they have been developed in the past in an established patient population to classify RA in order to be able to compare different patient populations.[9] This is the reason that these criteria are not the optimal instrument for the diagnosis of patients with an early RA.

Future developments

By means of new diagnostic procedures such as serological markers and advanced imaging methods such as ultrasound and magnetic resonance, new diagnostic criteria will be developed. This will make it possible to differentiate soon after the onset of symptoms between different inflammatory joint diseases with different presentations and disease courses.

Prognostic criteria

RA is not only a heterogeneous disease at presentation but the disease course itself is also highly variable and unpredictable. In combination with the inability to cure the disease despite the use of potentially toxic therapies, many attempts have been made to find prognostic factors that can correctly identify the course of the disease or the response to treatments. Although many prognostic factors have been identified, only a restricted number of factors appeared to be clinically relevant.[10,11] The only factor which is unquestionable is rheumatoid factor, which has been known about for more than a century. It is to be expected that through the intensive research in pharmacogenomics and proteomics new tests will become available in the near future which could be helpful in the diagnostic process. At the same time these tests will make it possible to predict the course of the disease in a particular patient as well as the response to the treatment. In this way the treatment of the patient with RA can be more tailormade: those with a bad prognosis could be treated from the start with the most effective (sometimes also the most expensive or toxic) agents. This will increase the effectiveness of the treatment enormously.

Therapeutic interventions

The interventions used in the treatment of RA can be divided into pharmacological and non-pharmacological modalities. As a cure of the disease is still not possible numerous non-pharmacological modalities are being applied in the management of patients with RA. They vary from occupational therapy to surgical synovectomy and from physical therapy and exercise to self-help educational programmes.[12] In the future, if it becomes possible to completely suppress the disease activity and cure the disease, the importance of these interventions will decrease.

The pharmacological interventions are conventionally divided into first and second line drugs. First line drugs include non-steroidal anti-inflammatory and COX-2 selective agents and do have a rapid suppressive effect on signs of inflammation without influencing the progression of the radiographic joint damage. Second line drugs, on the contrary, have a slow onset of action (from weeks up to months) and do slow down the progression of joint damage. The mechanism of action of these agents is largely unclear. As most of them had originally been developed for other diseases, in general by trial and error, it appeared that they had also beneficial effects in the treatment of RA (Table 4.1).

Next to the first and second line drugs, corticosteroids are being used both in a systemic (oral or parenteral) as well as in a local way

Table 4.1 Pharmacological treatment (second line drugs) effective in RA

Drug	Disease originally developed for
Parenteral gold	Tuberculoses
Hydroxychloroquine	Malaria
Chloroquine	
D-Penicillamine	Wilson disease
Sulfasalazine	Inflammatory bowel disease
Cytostatic drugs	Cancer
Cyclosporin	Organ transplantation
Methotrexate	Psoriasis

(intra-articular). Until around 1980 the pharmacotherapeutic strategy was rather conservative: first line drugs had to be given for months before second line agents were added. In cases where a second line agent was initiated, mostly the less toxic, least effective agent was chosen, or a very low dose of an effective drug was advised (go low, go slow principle). This strategy has changed dramatically and is now based on early suppression of the disease activity as soon as possible after the diagnosis of RA has been established, irrespective of the kind or number of drugs to be used.[13] As a result most of the RA patients are treated with at least two drugs and sometimes even up to seven or eight different drugs are concomitantly prescribed.

In the last decade, due to insights in the pathophysiology of the inflammatory process of RA, it became clear that the cytokines tumour necrosis factor alpha and interleukin 1 play an important role. Treatments were developed to specifically block these proinflammatory cytokines. Monoclonal antibodies or soluble receptors neutralising these cytokines are administered intravenously and subcutaneously to the patient.[14,15] These new treatments differ from the conventional second line agents in many ways: when given intravenously their onset of action is almost immediate, their mechanism of action is known and focussed, and the frequency of adverse reactions in the short term are low. However, the adverse reactions in the long term are as yet uncertain and therefore it is important to monitor these treatments for this aspect carefully.[16]

Future developments

In subsequent years the pharmacotherapeutic strategy will move from an aspecific broad approach to a tailormade target oriented approach.

Depending on the inflammatory and destructive profile of the patient anti-inflammatory drugs sometimes in combination with interventions that preserve or even repair cartilage and bone will be given.

Monitoring

The huge variety in disease expression in patients with RA has led in the past to the use of an enormous number of variables to monitor the disease course in daily clinical practice and to evaluate interventions in clinical trials. Many efforts have been taken in the past to standardise the assessment of RA, aiming at making study results interchangeable. Although a consensus has been reached over "what to assess" (Box 4.2), still further research is needed to improve the standardisation of the different methods.[17,18]

Box 4.2   Core set of variables assessed in RA clinical trials

- Number of tender joints
- Number of swollen joints
- Acute phase response
- Pain on Visual Analogue Scale
- Patient's global assessment of disease activity
- Physician's global assessment of disease activity
- Physical disability
- Radiographic studies

Due to the heterogeneity of the disease expression it is not possible to evaluate disease activity in all patients with RA with one single variable. Disease activity should be represented by a set of variables, which can be reported and analysed either separately or as part of an index of disease activity, for instance the disease activity score (DAS or DAS28).[19] For the evaluation of treatments in a clinical trial setting the currently two most frequently used criteria sets are the ACR 20% improvement criteria and the EULAR response criteria.[20,21] In addition remission criteria are available based on the absence of disease activity as measured by the disease activity score.

Daily clinical practice

In contrast to the global method of evaluation of the response to treatment, with most of the conventional drugs the need accurately to monitor disease activity also in daily clinical practice has been increasingly felt in the past years. The reason for this is the observation that with some of the conventional drugs, but in particular with the recent biological drugs, it is possible to titrate the treatment. Also, as we know that persistent disease activity causes many immediate problems to the patient it is important to suppress the disease activity of the patient as much as possible. In addition, it has been shown that this persistent disease activity is more likely to eventually lead to irreversible joint damage, a higher probability of the development of secondary lymphomas and even a reduction in life expectancy.[22–24] Disease controlling antirheumatic therapies do influence the disease activity, therefore to guide treatment decisions in an individual patient it is important to follow the fluctuating course of the disease activity as accurately as possible.[25] In fact this is not different from monitoring the glucose level in patients with diabetes mellitus and the blood pressure in patients with hypertension.

In daily clinical practice it is also important to know whether a patient is responding to an intervention, i.e. whether there is a significant/relevant change in disease activity (for instance ACR 20% response). In contrast with the clinical trials we are less interested in the exact amount/percentage of that response. The target of our treatment is not to obtain the highest possible percentage of improvement but to completely suppress the disease activity (remission), and if this is not conceivable to reach at least the lowest possible level. Therefore it is important to monitor the actual disease activity with a continuous variable like the disease activity score. For reasons of simplicity in daily clinical practice a minimal number of valid, not redundant, variables should be selected, therefore the DAS28 is being advocated. As the DAS28 is an easy to use, continuous disease activity measurement which is extensively validated in the clinical trial setting, this could be a valuable instrument for monitoring the disease course in daily clinical practice.

In previous studies the range of the DAS28 score has been calibrated against several clinical targets, which makes it possible to use this measurement as a titration instrument in daily clinical practice. A DAS28 level below 2.6 corresponds with being in remission according to the American Rheumatology Association criteria, a level below 3.2 represents low disease activity, between 3.2 and 5.1 moderate disease activity and above 5.1 high disease activity.[26,27,28] In addition it was shown that a change of 1.2 in an individual patient represents a statistically significant change. These two components (a significant change in disease activity and a target level) are important tools in the pharmacotherapeutic management of patients with RA. If the DAS28 is being measured at each visit it is possible to titrate the dose of the tumour necrosis factor alpha antagonist.

At the moment no treatments are available that directly influence the destruction of the joints apart from the disease activity, therefore the assessment of radiographic damage can be used to follow the disease course in the long term. The functional capacity as measured by patient questionnaires reflects a combination of the disease activity, radiographic damage and several other components and is therefore not suitable as an instrument to guide the therapy. Like x-rays, it is a useful instrument to monitor the disease course in the long term.

Future developments

The availability of more specific very effective treatments in the near future will stimulate the development of more precise instruments for evaluation. These instruments should be able to assess separately the different targets in the inflammatory process as well as the consequences of the disease process on the articular and extra-articular tissues. As in cardiology where the patient is being monitored wireless while being at home, also in rheumatology more and more emphasis will be placed on patient self-assessment. At home the patient can fill in questionnaires and even perform some simple blood tests and then send the results online to the rheumatologist who can advise the patient to adjust the treatments that he/she is using.

References

1 Statsny P. Association of the B-cell alloantigen DrW14 with rheumatoid arthritis. *N Engl J Med* 1978;**298**:869–71.
2 Deighton GM, Wentzel J, Cavanagh G *et al*. Contribution of inherited factors to rheumatoid arthritis. *Ann Rheum Dis* 1992;**51**:182–5.
3 Gregerson PK, Silver J, Winchester RJ. The shared epitope hypothesis – an approach to understanding the molecular genetics of susceptibility to rheumatoid arthritis. *Arthritis Rheum* 1987;**30**:1205–13.
4 De Jongh BM, van Romunde LKJ, Valkenberg HA, de Lange GG. Epidemiological study of HLA and GM in rheumatoid arthritis and related symptoms in an open Dutch population. *Ann Rheum Dis* 1984;**43**:613–9.
5 Thomson W, Harrison B, Ollier B *et al*. Quantifying the exact role of HLA-DRB1 alleles in susceptibility to inflammatory polyarthritis. *Arthritis Rheum* 1999;**42**:757–62.

6 Arnett FC, Edworthy SM, Bloch A *et al*. The American Rheumatism Association 1987 revised criteria for the classification of rheumatoid arthritis. *Arthritis Rheum* 1988;**31**:315–24.

7 Grahame R, Armstrong R, Simmons N *et al*. Chronic arthritis associated with the presence of intrasynovial rubella virus. *Ann Rheum Dis* 1983; **42**:2–4.

8 Steere AC, Grodzicki RL, Kornblatt AN *et al*. The spirochetal etiology of lyme disease. *N Engl J Med* 1983;**308**:733–6.

9 Harrison B, Symmons DPM, Barret EM, Silman AJ. The performance of the 1987 ARA classification criteria for rheumatoid arthritis in a population based cohort of patients with early inflammatory polyarthritis. *Br J Rheumatol* 1996;**35**:1096–1100.

10 Heijde van der DMFM, van Riel PLCM, Rijswijk van MH, Putte van de LBA. Influence of prognostic features on the final outcome in rheumatoid arthritis: a review of the literature. *Sem Arthritis Rheum* 1988;**17**:284–92.

11 Kroot EJA, Schellekens GA, Swinkels H *et al*. The prognostic value of the antiperinuclear factor, determined by a recently developed peptide-based ELISA, using anti citrulline-containing peptide antibodies (anti-CCP) in patients with recent-onset rheumatoid arthritis. *Arthitis Rheum* 2000;**43**: 1831–5.

12 Keysor JJ, Currey SS, Callahan LF. Behavioral aspects of arthritis and rheumatic disease self-management. *Dis Manage Health Outcomes* 2001;**9**:89–98.

13 Putte van de LBA, Gestel van AM, Riel van PLCM. Early treatment of rheumatoid arthritis: rationale, evidence, and implications. *Ann Rheum Dis* 1999;**57**:511–12.

14 Lipsky PE, Heijde van der DMFM, St Clair EW *et al*. Infliximab and methotrexate in the treatment of rheumatoid arthritis. *N Engl J Med* 2000;**343**:1594–602.

15 Bathon JM, Martin RW, Fleischmann RM *et al*. A comparison of etanercept and methotrexate in patients with early rheumatoid arthritis. *N Engl J Med* 2000;**343**:1586–93.

16 Finck B, Martin R, Fleischmann R, Moreland L, Schiff M, Bathon J. A phase III trial of etanercept vs methotrexate (MTX) in early rheumatoid arthritis (Enbrel ERA trial). *Arthritis Rheum* 1999;**42**(suppl.): S117 (abstract).

17 Silman A, Klareskog L, Breedveld F *et al*. Proposal to establish a register for the long term surveillance of adverse events in patients with rheumatic diseases exposed to biological agents: the EULAR Surveillance Register for Biological Compounds. *Ann Rhuem Dis* 2000;**59**:419–20.

18 Felson DT, Anderson JJ, Boers M *et al*. The American College of Rheumatology preliminary core set of disease activity measures for rheumatoid arthritis clinical trials. *Arthritis Rheum* 1993;**36**:729–40.

19 Van Riel PLCM. Provisional guidelines for measuring disease activity in clinical trials on rheumatoid arthritis. *Br J Rheumatol* 1992;**31**:793–6.

20 Prevoo MLL, Hof van't MA, Kuper HH, Leeuwen van MA, Putte van de LBA, Riel van PLCM. Modified disease activity scores that include twenty-eight-joint counts: development and validation in a prospective

longitudinal study of patients with rheumatoid arthritis. *Arthritis Rheum* 1995;**38**:44–8.

21 Gestel van AM, Prevoo MLL, Hof van't MA, Rijswijk MH, Putte van de LBA, Riel van PLCM. Development and validation of the European League Against Rheumatism response criteria for rheumatoid arthritis. Comparison with preliminary American College of Rheumatology and the World Health Organization/International League Against Rheumatism criteria. *Arthritis Rheum* 1996;**39**:34–40.
22 Gestel van AM, Anderson JJ, Riel van PLCM *et al.* ACR and EULAR improvement criteria have comparable validity in rheumatoid arthritis trials. *J Rheumatol* 1999;**26**:705–11.
23 Leeuwen van MA, Heijde van der DMFM, Rijswijk van MH *et al.* Interrelationship of outcome measures and process variables in early rheumatoid arthritis. *J Rheumatol* 1994;**21**:425–9.
24 Baecklund E, Ekbom A, Sparen P, Feltelius N, Klareskog L. Disease activity and risk of lymphoma in patients with rheumatoid arthritis: nested case-control study. *BMJ* 1998;**317**(7152):180–1.
25 Rasker JJ, Cosh JA. Cause and age at death in a prospective study of 100 patients with rheumatoid arthritis. *Ann Rheum Dis* 1981;**40**:115–20.
26 Heijde van der DM, Riel van PL, Nuver-Zwart HH, Gribnau FW, Putte van de LB. Effects of hydroxychloroquine and sulphasalazine on progression of joint damage in rheumatoid arthritis. *Lancet* 1989; **i**:1036–8.
27 Pinals RS, Masi AT, Larsen RA. Preliminary criteria for remission in rheumatoid arthritis. *Arthritis Rheum* 1981;**24**:1308–15.
28 Prevoo MLL, Gestel van AM, Hof van't MA, Rijswijk van MH, Putte van de LBA, Riel van PLCM. Remission in a prospective study of patients with rheumatoid arthritis. ARA preliminary remission criteria in relation to the disease activity score. *Br J Rheumatol* 1996;**35**:1101–5.

5: The future diagnosis and management of osteoarthritis

MICHAEL DOHERTY AND
STEFAN LOHMANDER

Osteoarthritis (OA) is by far the most common disorder to affect human joints. Its prevalence increases markedly with age such that it is a major cause of pain and disability in the elderly. The small joints of the hand, neck, low back and big toe are commonly affected but it is large joint OA of the knee and hip that causes the greatest community burden. Knee OA is more than five times more prevalent than hip OA, and together they affect 10–25% of people over the age of 65. In the developed world OA ranks fourth in health impact among women and eighth among men.[1] With the increasing proportion of elderly in these populations large joint OA of the knee and hip will become an even more important healthcare challenge in the future.

A current view of the nature of osteoarthritis

The traditional view of OA is that it is a degenerative disease of articular cartilage, the inevitable consequence of ageing, that once symptomatic always progresses, and for which nothing definitive can be done other than surgery. This pessimistic view is widely held not just by the general public but also by many of the healthcare professionals who manage patients with OA. In the last decade, however, it has become increasingly apparent that such a negative perspective is unfounded. For example:

- Study of the pathophysiology of OA shows it to be a metabolically active, dynamic process involving synthetic as well as degradative processes. Although there is localised loss of articular cartilage there is accompanying new tissue production, especially new bone, and adaptive remodelling of joint shape.[2]

- Much OA that is apparent on clinical or *x* ray examination remains clinically occult with no associated symptoms or functional impairment.[3,4]
- Although some people with symptomatic OA undoubtedly progress with worsening pain and continuing joint damage, many others have episodic symptoms and a good outcome even though their radiographic features may slowly continue to alter.
- There are a wide variety of effective non-pharmacological and drug interventions that can significantly reduce the pain and disability of OA.

A more appropriate view of OA is that it reflects the dynamic repair process of synovial joints (Figure 5.1).[5] It appears that a wide variety of insults may compromise or damage a joint. Often the initiating insult is unclear ("primary OA") but sometimes there is an obvious cause such as a torn ligament ("secondary OA"). The tissues that comprise a joint – cartilage, bone, synovium, capsule, ligament, muscle – depend on each other for their normal health and function. Insult to one tissue will impact on the others resulting in a common OA phenotype affecting the whole joint. The process of OA involves production of new bone, especially at the joint margin (osteophyte), thickening of the synovium and capsule, and remodelling of joint shape. Often the OA process can compensate for an insult, resulting in an anatomically altered but pain free functioning joint – "compensated OA". Sometimes, however, it fails, resulting in slowly

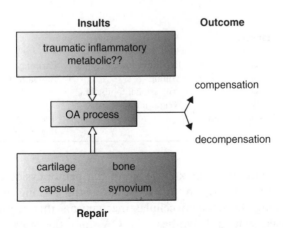

Figure 5.1 OA as a repair process to compensate for diverse damaging insults.

progressing damage with associated pain and impaired function, and eventual presentation as an OA patient with "joint failure". Such a perspective readily explains the marked clinical heterogeneity of OA and the variable outcomes observed.

Currently a number of risk factors are recognised that associate with the development of OA.[6] These risk factors vary at different joint sites (Table 5.1). They include constitutional factors, such as heredity, gender, ageing or obesity, and local mechanical factors such as trauma, instability and occupational and recreational usage. We also recognise some negative, possibly "protective" associations such as osteoporosis (hip OA) and smoking (knee OA). Risk factors for the development of OA may differ from those relating to the progression of OA (prognosis). For example, obesity and osteoporosis are minor risk factors for the development of hip OA but may be important risk factors for its more rapid progression.

Table 5.1 Risk factors for knee and hip OA

	Knee OA	Hip OA
Constitutional Risk factor		
Racial predisposition	All races	White individuals
Unidentified genetic factors	+++	+++
Heberden's nodes (fingers)	+++	+
Gender	Women > men	Women = men
Ageing	+++	++
Obesity	+++	+
Local		
Trauma	+++	+
Internal derangement	++	−
Instability	++	−
Occupation, recreation	Repetitive knee bending	Farming
	Mining	Elite athletes
	Professional footballing	
	Weight lifting	
Congenital/childhood joint disease	−	++ (e.g. dysplasia, Perthes)

However, although our knowledge of the pathophysiology of OA continues to expand, in 2001 we are still a long way from understanding the detailed cellular mechanisms that regulate joint tissue breakdown and synthesis in OA, and the ways in which recognised risk factors moderate its development and progression.

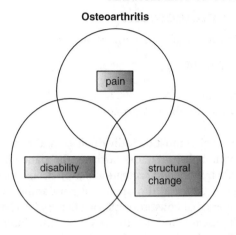

Figure 5.2 The loose correlation between pain, disability and structural change at the knee.

An important realisation in the last decade is that risk factors for pain and disability may differ from those for structural OA.[7,8] At the knee, for example, pain and disability correlate more strongly with muscle weakness, adverse psychosocial factors and obesity than with structural change (Figure 5.2). Again, the mechanisms for such correlation are unclear. Importantly, however, such observations have shifted the research focus not just to joint tissues other than cartilage but also to factors outside the joint. Increasing realisation that "knee pain is the malady, not OA"[4] has encouraged a more holistic approach to the study of regional musculoskeletal pain, with x ray evidence of OA a secondary rather than primary feature of interest. Inclusion of pain and disability within the research agenda of "OA" has extended the range of questions from:

- "what are the mechanisms of joint damage and repair in OA?" (joint tissue level), to
- "why do people get painful joints?" (person level), and from there to
- "what makes only some people seek help for their joint pain?" (society level).

The latter questions, of course, are of immediate relevance to clinical assessment and to healthcare delivery. Questions at all three levels, however, merit equal attention. They should be studied together, in parallel rather than in sequence.

Current management

The central objectives of management are to:

- educate the patient
- control pain
- optimise function
- beneficially modify the OA process.

Any management plan must be individualised and patient centred and take into account holistic factors such as the patient's daily activity requirements, their work and recreational aspirations, their perceptions and knowledge of OA, and the impact of pain and disability on their life.[9,10] The presence of constitutional risk factors for OA (e.g. obesity) and comorbid disease and its therapy will also influence decision making, as will the balance of safety and efficacy, patient preference, and the costs and local availability of individual treatments.

Although management is individualised there are currently evidence-based interventions,[9–11] largely life-style changes, that should be considered in all OA patients, especially those with large joint OA. These include:

- **Education**. Every doctor should inform their OA patients regarding the nature of their condition and its investigation, treatment and prognosis. However, in addition to being a professional responsibility, education itself improves outcome. Although the mechanisms are unclear, information access and therapist contact both reduce pain and disability of large joint OA, improve self-efficacy and reduce healthcare costs. Such benefits are modest but longlasting and safe.
- **Exercise**. Aerobic fitness training gives long-term reduction in pain and disability of large joint OA. It improves well being, encourages restorative sleep and benefits common comorbidity such as obesity, diabetes, chronic heart failure and hypertension. Local strengthening exercises for muscles acting over the knee and hip also reduce pain and disability from large joint OA with accompanying improvements in the reduced muscle strength, knee proprioception and standing balance that associate with knee OA. No age is exempt from receiving such a "prescription of activity".
- **Reduction of adverse mechanical factors**. For example, simple pacing of activities through the day and the use of shock-absorbing footwear and walking aids.

- **Advice on weight loss if obese.** There are epidemiological data, and some recent trial data, to show that reduction of obesity improves symptoms of large joint OA and may retard further structural progression.
- **Simple analgesia.** Paracetamol is the agreed oral drug of first choice and, if successful, is the preferred long term analgesic. This is because of its efficacy, lack of contraindications or drug interactions, long term safety, availability and low cost.

There are a wide variety of other non-pharmacological, drug and surgical interventions that may be considered additional options to be selected and added, as required, to these core interventions. These include:

- other oral agents – combined analgesics, non-steroidal anti-inflammatory drugs (NSAIDs), opioid analgesics, amitriptyline, and "nutripharmaceuticals" such as glucosamine and chondroitin sulphate
- topical creams – NSAIDs, capsaicin
- joint injections – steroid, hyaluronans, joint "washout"
- environmental modifications – such as a raised toilet seat, household aids
- other local physical treatments – including heat, cold, ultrasound, spa baths, patellar taping, knee braces
- surgical re-alignment (osteotomy).

The "final" option of course is surgical joint replacement. Although there are no universally applied criteria for surgery it is usually reserved for large joint OA patients with persistent severe pain and limitation despite adequate non-surgical treatment.

How strong is the current evidence for OA treatments?

Two groups recently reviewed the evidence for clinical trials for knee[9,10] and hip[10] OA in order to develop recommendations for management. The EULAR (European League Against Rheumatism) Task Force undertook a systematic review of intervention trials for knee OA published between 1966 and 1998.[9] They identified 680 trials investigating 23 treatment modalities. Most assessed drug treatments and over half were on non-steroidal anti-inflammatory drugs. Quality scores were in the low to mid range for most studies and few supplied enough data to permit calculation of the standardised effect size for the treatment. The Task Force concluded that randomised control trial evidence to guide treatment recommendations for knee OA is currently far from complete. The American College of Rheumatology Subcommittee on Osteoarthritis Guidelines undertook a less systematic review but included studies up to mid 2000.[10] These two groups came to similar conclusions as other evidence-based recent reviews[11,12] concerning the paucity of trial evidence, especially for non-pharmacological treatments of OA.

Such imbalance in research evidence in favour of drugs in part relates to greater difficulties in study design, for example with respect to patient blinding, for non-pharmacological compared to drug interventions. Predominantly, however, it reflects the investment and marketing requirements of the pharmaceutical industry.[13] The onus must therefore be on OA researchers, independent funding bodies and research ethics committees to prioritise research that addresses key questions in clinical management irrespective of the type of intervention involved.

Ways to improve future studies

In the last decade there has been a slow but steady improvement in the quality of clinical trials, not just in OA but in general. This probably reflects a more educated professional approach by clinical research groups, funding bodies, research ethics committees and journal editorial teams. It is apparent, however, that further progress is needed. In this decade we will hopefully see improvements both in study design and in the reporting of clinical trials that will enhance the quality and clinical relevance of the information obtained.[9,14] For example:

- **More consistency in outcome measures**. The use of a smaller number of well validated instruments that assess core outcomes such as pain and disability will facilitate comparison of data between studies and the pooling of data for systematic reviews and meta-analyses.[14]
- **Longer duration of study**. Most studies are relatively short term (6 weeks to 6 months) and only a handful extend to 1–2 years. Many OA patients require treatment over many years and long term efficacy data are clearly required. Long periods of study are also essential for the assessment of any modification of joint structure.

- **Inclusion of a broader spectrum of patients and examination of predictors of response**. Often particular patient characteristics such as old age, severe x ray change, presence of knee effusion or obesity are considered exclusions for clinical trials. This is on the assumption, rather than the knowledge, that such factors influence treatment outcome. Study of homogeneous trial populations (e.g. patients aged 45–70, not obese, no comorbidity, all with mild to moderate x ray change) has the advantage of reducing the number of patients that need to be studied. However, it severely limits the generalisability of the findings obtained. An alternative approach is to include a larger number of more representative patients who vary in their clinical characteristics.[15] Randomisation will result in equally varied subjects in each of the trial groups and the specific clinical variables can then be examined as possible predictors of response. When this has been done the result is often contrary to preconceived opinion; for example, the presence of clinically assessed inflammation at the knee does not influence response to oral non-steroidal anti-inflammatory drugs or intra-articular injection of steroids.[9] Knowledge of clinical predictors is important since they may guide clinical management decisions.
- **Factorial design**.The evidence for most interventions relates to their use as single therapy. In the "real world", however, management plans include several treatments given concurrently. More use of a factorial design in clinical trials would permit efficient examination of combinations of treatment and explore the possibility of additive benefits of two or more interventions.
- **Fuller reporting of trial data**. Recent widespread adoption of the CONSORT agreement for more uniform reporting of clinical trials[16] should improve the quality and transparency of trial reports. Also the increasing use of website publishing, with extended trial data on the internet but summary data in the article, should improve the availability and assessment of trial data.

Development areas with potential major impact for the future

Investigation of basic pathophysiology

Better understanding of the normal physiology of joint tissues, their response to insult (biochemical, mechanical, immunological) and the alterations apparent in OA joints will give us better insight into the detailed mechanisms that are involved. Such knowledge may then open up new avenues of intervention for both symptom control and slowing or even halting of progressive structural change.

There is a considerable ongoing effort in these basic areas of research, involving expertise and techniques from many varied disciplines. The search, in general, is for informative "surrogate markers" of OA. Such markers may give us information on diagnosis (even before the establishment of obvious, irreversible structural change), current activity of the OA process, or prognosis (Figure 5.3). Individual markers could give information on one, two or all three of these. At our present stage of knowledge it is clinical markers that give us most information in all three respects. However, various imaging modalities, especially magnetic resonance imaging, offer the possibility of more sensitive assessment of joint physiology and structure and thus assistance in early diagnosis, assessment of further structural change and insight into OA physiology. Measurement of biochemical markers in blood, urine or knee joint fluid may also detect abnormal degradation and/or synthesis of joint tissues and thus assist in the early diagnosis of OA, the assessment of current activity, and the response of OA joints to treatments that may modify disease outcome. Surrogate markers of OA, whether based on structural or metabolic change, will probably find use first in "proof-of-concept" clinical trials aimed at disease modification in OA.

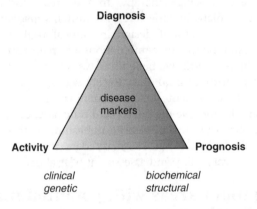

Figure 5.3 Markers of OA.

However, probably the main area that promises the greatest impact in terms of insight into OA in the next 10 years is genetics. The strong heritability of nodal generalised OA (Heberden's nodes of distal finger joints and tendency to OA of knees and other joints) has been known for half a century. In the last decade it has become increasingly apparent that knee OA and hip OA also have a strong genetic component.[17,18] The search for specific genes that associate with OA was stimulated by identification of mutations in the gene (COL2A1) that encodes type II collagen, a major protein in articular cartilage, in rare families in which half the offspring have atypical, young onset OA in association with other skeletal abnormalities.[19] Mutations of COL2A1 have not been found in common larger joint OA, but study of such single gene (monogenic) disorders fuelled the more difficult search for genetic associations in common OA. OA is a "common complex disorder" in which multiple genetic and environmental factors interact in different combinations to result in a similar clinical phenotype. Unlike monogenic disease where a rare mutation of just a single gene always causes disease, common variations of many genes are involved each with perhaps only a relatively small risk of OA contributed by each gene. Like other risk factors, these may differ according to joint site, and relate to either the development or progression of OA. The approximate location of several genes that associate with hand, knee or hip OA are now being identified from the study of families who have at least two affected siblings. While searching for these genes, it is important to recognise that the inheritance of for example a particular structural feature on an x ray image of a joint may not be the same as that for severe symptomatic OA leading to joint replacement. The technology of gene identification is rapidly advancing and within the next decade it is likely that we will know the genes and their predisposing variants. Individual genes might only exert an effect in a particular joint if other genetic, constitutional or environmental risk factors are present (Figure 5.4). Therefore, once predisposing genes are identified, the next stage will be gene–gene and gene–environmental interaction studies to determine the mechanisms by which predisposition occurs.

Much attention is currently given by the pharmaceutical industry to the principle of "disease modification" in OA. Disease modification in OA might lead to the preservation and/or regeneration of joint structure. The accompanying hypothesis states that this would also lead in the long term to preserved or improved function and decreased pain. At this time, both these aspects of disease modification in OA remain unproven. Ongoing research on the detailed mechanisms of cartilage and joint biochemistry and physiology, along with the accelerating rate of genetic discovery, will no doubt increase the number of potential treatment targets in OA, putting great pressure on our methods to monitor clinical trials of these new disease targets.

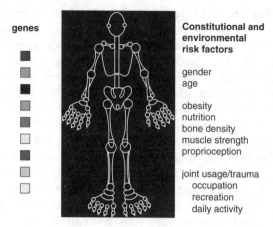

genes

Constitutional and
environmental
risk factors

gender
age

obesity
nutrition
bone density
muscle strength
proprioception

joint usage/trauma
occupation
recreation
daily activity

Figure 5.4 Multiple genes, constitutional and environmental risk factors combine in different ways to produce OA at specific joint sites. Future study of the way in which genes and other risk factors interrelate will inform about the mechanisms involved.

The accompaniment to genetic discovery work is the continuing identification of further risk factors. Physiological factors that have only recently begun to be studied include muscle strength, joint position sense (proprioception), lower limb balance, joint stability and biomechanical alignment.[20–22] We know that the assessment of all current known risk factors for OA does not explain the totality of OA observed, so it is likely that other factors that relate to dysfunction in OA have yet to be identified. The advantage of a total genome screen for OA genes is that it may elucidate such unknown risk factors. Many researchers expect that genes relating to known structural components of cartilage are the principal candidates to explain the genetic component of OA. However, it may be that unsuspected changes in other tissues (for example bone, capsule, muscle) turn out to be as, if not more, important in the pathogenesis of OA structural change.

The better understanding of pain mechanisms in general could also lead to improved treatment of chronic OA pain. We still have incomplete knowledge of the complex processing and modulation of sensory input from pain nerve fibres, particularly with respect to chronic pain perception. The current search for novel analgesic agents that alone or in combination influence pain pathways at different central nervous system sites (peripheral, spinal cord, higher centres) may improve the treatment options for OA as much as for other chronic pain states. In particular the requirement is for effective but safe agents for moderate to severe pain. It is also likely that methods to widen the applicability and impact of non-pharmacological approaches to chronic pain and "coping" will be forthcoming. Included in this is the more formal harnessing of the placebo response that is such a marked feature in OA clinical trials.

Improved application of current knowledge

The vast majority of people with large joint OA are managed in primary care by self-management and advice from general practitioners, pharmacists and allied health professionals. Although there are scant data on the quality of care for such people, it appears that many receive suboptimal or even inappropriate treatment and advice, especially with respect to education and lifestyle modification. This is probably also true for those who proceed to secondary care. Improved awareness, knowledge and interest in OA and subsequent wider application of current treatment strategies would make a major impact on the community burden of OA. This contrasts with the common misconception that only novel treatment "breakthroughs" can help someone with OA. If better treatments, or even "breakthroughs", for OA were to become available, appropriate education of healthcare professionals and efficient delivery of such treatments will still be required. The situation with gout, another chronic locomotor condition, is salutary. We have excellent understanding of the pathogenesis of gout and effective treatments to prevent the formation of the causative urate crystals. It is one of the few rheumatic diseases in which the aim of management is "cure". Regrettably, however, people correctly diagnosed with gout often persist for years with poorly controlled and undertreated disease. Irrespective of any future advances in OA management, appropriate education of healthcare professionals will always remain a priority. Given its high prevalence and impact, knowledge of large joint OA and its management should always be prominent in the training curriculum of general practitioners and allied health professionals.

Developments in surgery

Surgical interventions for large joint OA include joint debridement, osteotomies and joint replacements. Cartilage repair as currently practised is an experimental treatment for joint cartilage damage in the younger individual, but not for OA.[23] Evidence for the effectiveness of debridement as a treatment for OA is ambiguous.[24]

Osteotomy is mainly used for knee OA in the young and active individual to realign the loading axis from a diseased medial joint compartment to the usually more intact lateral compartment. It may significantly delay or prevent the need for a joint replacement.[23]

Joint replacement is an effective treatment for OA patients with severe symptoms and/or severe joint destruction.[25,26] Notwithstanding this statement, much effort is being spent to improve several aspects of this treatment. Implant component wear and mechanical loosening are focus areas for research: it is hoped that further improvements in implant materials and design will decrease wear rates and the formation of wear particles. A decrease in wear particles may lessen the risk for implant loosening. Implant fixation may be improved by the introduction of new material surface properties, as well as by the treatment of at risk individuals with drugs such as bisphosphonates or parathyroid hormone. Improvements in these areas will be especially important for the young and active individuals who need a joint replacement but who are at the highest risk for implant loosening and wear.

While much attention is given to these "technical" aspects of joint surgery, much less is given to the appropriate selection of patients for joint replacement. Thus, we are still somewhat ignorant with regard to the characteristics of "responders" and "non-responders" to joint surgery, and few systematic studies have been performed. This is an area in which improved understanding might provide as great a gain in overall effectiveness as the technical improvements mentioned.

Strategies for primary prevention

Strategies to reduce the incidence of large joint OA have been suggested.[6] Successful reduction of modifiable risk factors such as obesity (especially for knee OA in women) and occupational and recreational joint trauma could significantly reduce the incidence and delay the age of onset of large joint OA. Increase in the amount of regular physical activity undertaken by the community could also retard age-associated decline in muscle strength, knee proprioception and balance[27,28] and delay decompensation of the OA process. Such lifestyle modifications relating to weight, exercise and trauma avoidance are relevant to the health of other body systems and should lead to concurrent improvements in the incidence and severity of cardiovascular disease, stroke and maturity onset diabetes.

The practical problem, of course, is effecting such lifestyle changes in large numbers of people. As has been learnt from antismoking and antiobesity campaigns, simply informing individuals about possible health consequences does not readily lead to modification of habitual behaviour. There are different stages of "willingness to change"[29] and it is only if an individual really does want to change that he or she is likely to do so. Encouraging people to shift towards that important stage of willingness is problematical. One approach is to increase the relevance of the lifestyle change to the individual in question. For example, everyone is at some risk of developing hip OA. But if the sibling of a person who has undergone joint replacement for hip OA is informed that he or she is seven times more likely to develop hip OA him or herself (because of this genetic exposure) he or she may be more inclined to consider lifestyle changes to reduce that risk. Such selective targeting of people at special risk has not been attempted. At present, subjects who are at special risk of large joint OA may be identified by:

- an overt family history of large joint OA
- presence of multiple Heberden's nodes (increased risk of knee OA in the sixties and seventies)
- presence of unilateral large joint OA (increased risk of developing contralateral large joint OA)
- previous knee meniscus or ligament injury
- occupational or recreational repetitive overusage.

Such individuals might prove more amenable to lifestyle advice if they are informed of their risk. The concept of risk, however, can be difficult to explain. Often it is confounded by anecdotal observation, for example by having an overweight, underactive uncle who lived to 95 without any knee OA. Nevertheless, the discovery of genes that predispose to large joint OA and their profiling within individuals may prove more persuasive. Examination for predisposing genes from a simple blood test combined with the assessment of modifiable risk factors may permit more accurate determination of individual risk and more specific recommendation for lifestyle change. Such genetic profiling might be undertaken simultaneously for all common complex disorders. If predisposing genes are present for several conditions, including those that shorten life, the rationale for appropriate lifestyle modification may be more meaningful.

The application of genetic discovery, of course, may extend beyond their use as markers for OA. For example "gene therapy" may allow selective targeting of drugs to certain tissues within OA joints, avoiding effects and potential toxicity in non-OA tissues. The possibility of intervening in the expression or functioning of predisposing genes and their products may also prove possible. These authors, however, believe that such advances will follow at a much later date than the more practical and already foreseeable issues listed above. Whatever happens, the next few decades should prove a most informative and exciting time for the better understanding and treatment of large joint OA.

Summary

Osteoarthritis (OA) is the most prevalent form of arthritis and a major cause of disability in the elderly. Contrary to popular opinion, OA is a metabolically dynamic process, representing an enhancement of the inherent degradation and repair process of joints. Diverse genetic, constitutional and environmental risk factors are recognised. Factors that predispose to structural change differ from those for pain and disability. A number of effective non-pharmacological, drug and surgical interventions are currently available. Advances in imaging techniques and in biochemical markers are expected to improve earlier diagnosis and monitoring of disease progression. However, it is study of the genetic predisposition to OA that is predicted to result in the greatest advances in our understanding of OA pathogenesis. The current management of OA is often suboptimal and an improved awareness and education of healthcare professionals will result in major benefits in management. Lifestyle modifications to reduce risk factors for OA (reduction in obesity, increased activity, avoidance of joint trauma) could have a major impact on reducing the incidence and severity of large joint OA, as well as benefiting common diseases in other body systems. Despite practical difficulties, strategies to effect such primary and secondary prevention of OA should receive priority for implementation, especially with the increasing proportion of elderly in the population.

References

1 Murray CJL, Lopez AD. *The global burden of disease*. Geneva: World Health Organization, 1997.
2 Hammerman D. The biology of osteoarthritis. *New Engl J Med* 1989;**320**: 1322–30.

3 Davis MA, Ettinger WH, Neuhaus JM, Barclay JD, Segal MR. Correlates of knee pain among US adults with and without radiographic knee osteoarthritis. *J Rheumatol* 1992;**19**:1943–9.

4 Hadler NM. Knee pain is the malady – not osteoarthritis. *Ann Intern Med* 1992;**116**:598–9.

5 Radin EL, Burr DB. Hypothesis: joints can heal. *Sem Arthritis Rheum* 1984;**13**:293–302.

6 Felson D, Zhang Y. An update on the epidemiology of knee and hip osteoarthritis with a view to prevention. *Arthritis Rheum* 1998;**41**:1343–55.

7 Van Baar ME, Dekker J, Lemmens JAM, Oostendorp RAB, Bijlsma WJ. Pain and disability in patients with osteoarthritis of hip or knee: the relationship with articular, kinesiological and psychological characteristics. *J Rheumatol* 1998;**25**:125–33.

8 Creamer P, Lethbridge-Cejku M, Hochberg MC. Factors associated with functional impairment in symptomatic knee osteoarthritis. *Rheumatology* 2000;**39**:490–6.

9 Pendleton A, Arden N, Dougados M *et al*. EULAR recommendations for the management of knee osteoarthritis: report of a task force of the Standing Committee for International Studies Including Therapeutic Trials (ESCISIT). *Ann Rheum Dis* 2000;**59**:936–44.

10 American College of Rheumatology Subcommittee on Osteoarthritis Guidelines. Recommendations for the medical management of osteoarthritis of the hip and knee. 2000 update. *Arthritis Rheum* 2000;**43**:1905–15.

11 Walker-Bone K, Javaid K, Arden N, Cooper C. Medical management of osteoarthritis. *BMJ* 2000;**321**:936–40.

12 Dieppe P, Chard J, Faulkner A, Lohmander S. Osteoarthritis. In: Godlee F, ed. *Clinical Evidence. A compendium of the best evidence for effective health care*. London: BMJ Publishing Group, 2000: Issue 4. http://www.evidence.org/.

13 Chard JA, Tallon D, Dieppe PA. Epidemiology of research into interventions for the treatment of osteoarthritis of the knee joint. *Ann Rheum Dis* 2000;**59**:414–18.

14 A task force of the Osteoarthritis Research Society. Design and conduct of clinical trials in patients with osteoarthritis. *Osteoarthritis Cart* 1996;**4**:217–43.

15 Doherty M, Jones A. Design of clinical trials in knee osteoarthritis: practical issues for debate. *Osteoarthritis Cart* 1998;**6**:371–3.

16 Begg CB, Cho M, Eastwood S *et al*. Improving the quality of reporting of randomised controlled trials. The CONSORT statement. *JAMA* 1996;**276**:637–9.

17 Spector TD, Cicuttini F, Baker J, Loughlin J, Hart D. Genetic influences on osteoarthritis in women: a twin study. *BMJ* 1996;**312**:940–4.

18 Lanyon P, Muir K, Doherty S, Doherty M. Assessment of a genetic contribution to osteoarthritis of the hip: sibling study. *BMJ* 2000;**321**:1179–83.

19 Jimenez S, Williams CJ, Karasick D. Hereditary osteoarthritis. In: Brandt K, Doherty M, Lohmader S, eds. *Osteoarthritis*. Oxford: Oxford University Press, 1998;31–49.

20 Slemenda C, Brandt KD, Heilman DK *et al.* Quadriceps weakness and osteoarthritis of the knee. *Ann Intern Med* 1997;**127**:97–104.
21 Pai Y-C, Rymer WZ, Chang RW, Sharma L. Effect of age and osteoarthritis on knee proprioception. *Arthritis Rheum* 1997;**40**:2260–5.
22 Sharma L, Hayes KW, Felson DT *et al.* Does laxity alter the relationship between strength and physical function in knee osteoarthritis? *Arthritis Rheum* 1999;**42**:25–32.
23 Buckwalter JA, Lohmander LS. Surgical approaches to preserving and restoring cartilage. In: Brandt KD, Doherty M, Lohmander LS, eds. *Osteoarthritis*. Oxford: Oxford University Press, 1998;378–88.
24 Ike RW. Joint lavage. In: Brandt KD, Doherty M, Lohmander LS, eds. *Osteoarthritis*. Oxford: Oxford University Press, 1998;359–77.
25 Knutson K. Arthroplasty and its complications. In: Brandt KD, Doherty M, Lohmander LS, eds. *Osteoarthritis*. Oxford: Oxford University Press, 1998; 388–402.
26 Dieppe P, Basler HD, Chard J *et al.* Knee replacement surgery for osteoarthritis: effectiveness, practice variations, indications and possible determinants of utilization. *Rheumatology (Oxford)* 1999;**38**:73–83.
27 Ettinger WH, Burns R, Messier SP *et al.* A randomised trial comparing aerobic exercise and resistance exercise with a health education program in older adults with knee osteoarthritis. *JAMA* 1997;**277**:25–31.
28 Messier SP, Royer TD, Craven TE *et al.* Long-term exercise and its effect on balance in older, osteoarthritic adults: results from the Fitness, Arthritis, and Seniors Trial (FAST). *J Am Geriatr Soc* 2000;**48**:131–8.
29 Prochaska JO, DiClemente CC, Norcross JC. In search of how people change. *Am Psychol* 1992;**47**:1102–14.

Recommended reading

Brandt K, Doherty M, Lohmander S, eds. *Osteoarthritis*. Oxford: Oxford University Press, 1998 (second edition, 2002).
Young A, Harries M, eds. *Physical Activity for Patients. An Exercise Prescription.* London: Royal College of Physicians of London, 2001.

6: The future diagnosis and management of osteoporosis

DONNCHA O'GRADAIGH AND
JULIET COMPSTON

Introduction

... an old lord, Aegyptius, stooped with age (Homer's Odyssey)

It is often the concerted efforts of industry, political will, healthcare professionals and their patients that lead to delivery of better health from bench to bedside and beyond to the community. The World Health Organization has identified this decade for particular attention to the disorders of bones and joints, and osteoporosis will be at the forefront of these efforts. This chapter will highlight controversial issues in its diagnosis and management and consider alternatives currently under evaluation. Scientific theories and developments in these areas, and the broader developments that can be anticipated in the global delivery of care will also be considered.

Investing in the future – research evidence

Critical appraisal of the medical research evidence is an essential part of therapeutic decision making, allocation of resources, and is important to attract the consumer's confidence. Expert consensus opinion is valuable in formulating guidelines for practice – "knowledge, to become wisdom, requires experience" (Corrigan). The World Health Organization, the National Institute of Health in the US and the International Osteoporosis Foundation have published their deliberations in the last year, as have the Royal College of Physicians together with the Bone and Tooth Society in the UK. In the UK, a National Institute for Clinical Excellence has been established by the government to provide evidence-based recommendations. It is highly improbable, and indeed undesirable,

Table 6.1 Currently available evidence for interventions in osteoporosis (adapted with permission of the Royal College of Physicians, London from Writing Group of the Bone and Tooth Society of Great Britain and the Royal College of Physicians[1])

Selected drugs	Postmenopausal bone loss reduction	Fracture risk reduction		
		Spine	Hip	Others
Alendronate	A	A	A	A
Calcitonin	A	A	B	B
Calcitriol	A	A	A	ND
Calcium and Vitamin D	A	ND	A	A
Etidronate	A	A	B	B
Hormone replacement therapy	A	A	A	B
Raloxifene (SERM)	A	A	ND	ND
Risedronate	A	A	A	A

ND = no effect demonstrated.

Grade A = meta-analysis or at least one randomised controlled trial or well designed controlled study without randomisation; Grade B = at least one well-designed other trial type (cohort, case-control or quasi-experimental study); Grade C = expert opinion, clinical experience of authorities.

that a body advising those who ultimately control healthcare resources would not include cost effectiveness in its overall analysis (otherwise merely duplicating work already available from other bodies, such as the Cochrane Collaboration).

All of these organisations use a standard classification of research evidence (Table 6.1). In the context of osteoporosis, effects on bone mineral density and fracture risk must be considered separately. Evidence for the latter requires larger studies over an extended period, and therefore relatively few interventions have a high grade of evidence in this setting. A number of outstanding issues need to be considered, including:

- Variations between populations have been recognised in areas such as genetics and bone mass – as most trials have studied Caucasians, they must be interpreted with caution before global strategies are considered.
- Outcomes should include robust estimates of number needed to treat, as this reflects effectiveness (the product of efficacy and

compliance), and the rate at which the adverse event occurs without intervention.

- The number of people sustaining a fracture is a more appropriate end-point than the number of fractures (as one fracture increases the risk of another irrespective of intervention).
- Specific groups should be identified for whom more cost effective short term treatment strategies can be designed.
- Low cost, high compliance interventions (even of modest efficacy) may offer greater *cost* effectiveness than a high cost, low compliance strategy (even if of greater efficacy).

The diagnosis of osteoporosis

Osteoporosis is defined in pathological terms as "a progressive systemic disease characterised by low bone density and microarchitectural deterioration of bone tissue, with a consequent increase in bone fragility and susceptibility to fracture". However, this fragility and susceptibility may only result in an osteoporotic fracture (a vertebral fracture or minimal trauma fracture at another site, in the absence of alternative pathology) if there is a convergence of environmental factors, other illness and circumstances leading to falls (Figure 6.1). Osteoporosis is "established" once such a fracture occurs. While this is certainly unambiguous, osteoporosis should ideally be identified before a fracture has occurred. Therefore, for practical purposes, measured bone mineral density is compared to a

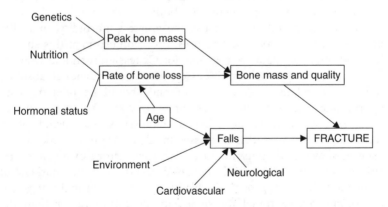

Figure 6.1 Multiple factors contribute to the overall risk of fractures.

reference peak bone mass and expressed as a T-score. Osteoporosis is then defined as a T-score of -2.5 or less, the threshold at which the absolute risk of fracture is "high". Using this classification, the disease therefore "occurs" at a selected point in a continuous slope of declining bone density.

Measurement of bone mineral density

Measurements of bone mineral density are currently most commonly obtained using dual energy x ray absorptiometry, for which there are internationally recommended indications. Current limitations of this technique include:

- Limited reference ranges for males, younger patients and different ethnic groups.
- Scoliosis, other deformities and degenerative changes (osteophytes, sclerosis, extraskeletal calcification) in the spine result in spurious increases in bone density when using anteroposterior spine views.
- The working definition of osteoporosis is not related to any definitive pathological event; therefore, definitions of bone mineral density of significant risk may need to be site specific.
- The role of bone mineral density in monitoring the efficacy of treatment is currently unclear; accurate ascertainment of response may require up to three or more years of therapy.

It has recently been suggested that for diagnostic purposes, total hip bone mineral density should be regarded as the gold standard since this measurement is predictive of both cervical and trochanteric fractures, which collectively cause the greatest morbidity, mortality and cost of all osteoporotic fractures. Precision errors at this site are low and reference data are available for Caucasian men and women. For the purposes of fracture risk assessment in an individual, absolute rather than relative risk is relevant and should be related to an appropriate time interval, for example 10 years. Measurements of bone mineral density at other skeletal sites and using other technologies are useful in risk assessment, as are other risk factors such as previous fragility fracture, maternal history of hip fracture, risk factors for falling and increased levels of bone markers of resorption. This approach is likely to be increasingly used to determine interventional thresholds in the future rather than the T-score definition of osteoporosis.

Recognising previous fractures

Past or prevalent fractures increase the risk of further fracture, ranging from a 3- to 12-fold increased risk of hip or vertebral fracture, respectively, in the presence of one or more previous vertebral deformities. Although 60% of vertebral fractures may be clinically unrecognised, routine assessment to determine the presence of such fractures is not current practice. Morphometric x ray absorptiometry utilises lateral images obtained at the same time as densitometric assessment, increasing scanning costs and time. While this has a number of theoretical and practical advantages over conventional radiography in the detection of spinal fractures, reservations concerning reference ranges and correctly recognising other causes of vertebral deformity (such as degenerative changes or Scheuermann's disease) have limited the use of this technique to date. At present, many individuals presenting to accident & emergency or orthopaedic services with fragility fractures are not referred for appropriate investigation and treatment; correcting this deficit is an important priority for the future.

Biochemical markers of bone turnover

A person's bone density at a point in time is the product of the rate at which bone density is lost and the peak density attained at skeletal maturity (Figure 6.2). Biochemical assessment of osteoporosis is not yet in reach, though markers of bone formation and resorption (Table 6.2) are currently under intense investigation. Some markers correlate with rates of change in bone mineral density, and others have been shown to accurately predict fractures in the elderly. However, ongoing difficulties include:

- biovariability in the "normal" ranges (i.e. variations within an individual from day to day or during one day).
- variance in the laboratory measurement of these markers (i.e. obtaining the same result when repeatedly testing the same sample).
- identifying a sufficiently sensitive and specific single test or combination of tests.

However, as methodology improves it is likely that bone turnover markers will add to the overall assessment of osteoporosis and may eventually influence treatment decisions.

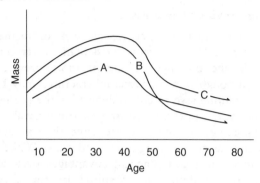

Figure 6.2 Reduced bone mass in later life may occur due to a low peak being attained (A), or due to accelerated loss (B), compared with normal peak and rate of loss (C).

Table 6.2 Biochemical markers of bone turnover

Resorption	Formation
Urinary pyridinoline	Serum bone specific alkaline phosphatase
Urinary deoxypyridinoline	Serum osteocalcin
Serum C-terminal cross-linked telpopetide of type I collagen (C1PT)	Serum C-terminal propeptide of type I procollagen (P1CP)
Urine C-terminal cross-linked telopeptide of type I collagen (CTx)	Serum N-terminal propeptide of type I procollagen (P1NP)
Urine N-terminal cross-linked telopeptide of type I collagen (NTx)	
Serum tartrate-resistant acid phosphatase (TRAP)	

The assessment of bone microarchitecture

A mighty maze, but not without a plan! (Alexander Pope, *Essay on Man*)

Microarchitectural deterioration disrupts the structural framework of cancellous bone. However, it is not possible to directly measure this *in vivo*. High resolution magnetic resonance imaging of the wrist can assess the cancellous structure, but long scanning times, relatively expensive equipment and the need for expert interpretation of the images preclude the routine use of this technique. Quantitative computed tomography enables measurement of volumetric bone density and separate evaluation of cancellous and cortical bone, and also has the potential to assess cancellous bone structure. This can be applied to the vertebrae (axial quantitative computed tomography) or to peripheral sites (peripheral quantitative computed tomography). While radiation dose in peripheral quantitative computed tomography is quite low, it is unacceptably high in axial quantitative computed tomography for routine clinical use. Furthermore, scanning times are long, and accessibility is limited.

Ultrasonography, in use for many years in materials engineering, assesses material elasticity (Young's modulus) and is related to mineral density and bone architecture – sound propagates more quickly through more dense, intact structures. Expressed as broadband ultrasound attenuation (in dB/MHz) and as speed of sound (in m/s), both values are used in a "stiffness index". Sound waves must also travel through adjacent soft tissue, and for this and other reasons the calcaneus (heel) is commonly used. Broadband ultrasound attenuation and speed of sound can predict fracture as accurately as BMD, though each detects different aspects of the overall susceptibility to fracture. However, several problems remain to be resolved before both these values can be reliably used for screening or intervention purposes. Ultrasound technology is still grappling with variability between various machines, and with imprecision of measurements. Patient factors (variability in skin temperature, ultrasound beam attenuation at the skin surface, variation in soft-tissue thickness and density) also pose problems. Technological advances (coupling gels, uniformity in sound wave focussing, software to handle soft tissue artefact) are expected to overcome many of these limitations. Being portable, non-ionising and inexpensive, and as ultrasound machines are already widely available to the public, this will have a considerable impact on patterns of self-referral. Unfortunately, commercialisation is likely to hamper future research efforts, particularly in trying to achieve standardisation and improved reliability of measurements across various providers. The clinical value of ultrasound in the future therefore remains uncertain.

Genetic influences

Genetic factors account for 60–80% of the observed variation in bone mineral density. Osteoporosis is polygeneic (many different genes contributing) and involves a complex interaction between genetic inheritance and the environment (including nutrition, general health, exposure to drugs, etc.). Associations between bone mineral density and, in some studies fracture, and a number of polymorphisms (variations in the DNA sequence within a gene) have been identified. These are reviewed in detail elsewhere, but the following observations are of interest with respect to future developments:

- Polymorphisms in the collagen type I gene (*COLIA1*) and the gene for transforming growth factor beta (*TGF-β*) have been directly associated with both bone mineral density and fracture risk.
- Several polymorphisms in the vitamin D receptor gene have been identified and associations with bone mineral density reported, although these findings have not always been consistent. There is also evidence that polymorphisms in this gene may affect the response to vitamin D and calcium supplementation.
- Polymorphisms in genes for other key regulatory growth factors are currently being investigated.

Although the human genome has been recently published, searches at new sites will probably be driven by fresh discoveries in bone biology rather than the reverse. However, one can foresee that as this technology becomes more accessible, individuals will be screened for genetic variations predisposing to a variety of common diseases, perhaps driven by the health insurance sector. In future, single or multiple genetic variations may well aid in the identification of those most at risk, but overall risk assessment, incorporating other factors as discussed above, will continue to be required for treatment.

If you know any better methods than these, be frank and tell them; if not, use these with me. (Horace)

The management of osteoporosis

The management of osteoporosis raises issues that are unique to bone and joint diseases. For most people there is a considerable period between the age at which osteoporosis may be detected and that at which most fractures occur. Many people who fracture will not have osteoporosis, while others with osteoporosis will not fracture. This has considerable implications for therapeutic decisions, and for the allocation of resources. The latter will also be affected by differences between society's (typically utilitarian) perspective and that of the individual increasingly empowered by the information age and directly targeted in the future by pharmaceutical advertising.

In looking towards the future management of osteoporosis, one can anticipate changes in the patient selection for treatment, in the use of current therapies and in the development of novel agents, together with increasing emphasis on cost effectiveness and on reducing the number of people developing osteoporosis. In the words of Ernest Rutherford, "we haven't got the money, so we've got to think!"

Screening

Screening is appropriate for a common disease, which has a significant impact on the population's health, for which a highly effective treatment is available and for which a definitive and accurate test is available and acceptable. A distinction must be made between formally testing all members of a population (screening) and selecting a particular subgroup for testing (case finding). The latter reflects the approach currently recommended in osteoporosis.

A large proportion of those identified by questionnaire-based case findings have normal bone density and this is therefore not a suitable tool to select for bone mass measurement. Computer based expert systems (artificial neural networks) allow large amounts of data (an increased number of questions and response categories) to be rapidly analysed. However, a recent example failed to achieve any substantial improvement over more simple dichotomous variables or categories.

Developments in current therapies

Developments will be driven by the need for drugs that have a rapid onset of fracture prevention, prolonged benefit after cessation of treatment (referred to as offset of action), and high effectiveness and compliance. In particular, there is considerable interest in the development of anabolic agents to improve bone quality in those already at high risk.

Hormonal therapies

Observations of accelerated bone loss in the early postmenopausal years make hormone replacement therapy a rational approach to the treatment for osteoporosis. However, evidence of anti-fracture efficacy largely comes from observational studies (which tend to overestimate the treatment effect as those who choose to take hormone replacement therapy are healthier for other reasons).

Furthermore, there is increasing evidence that the beneficial skeletal effects of hormone replacement therapy are not maintained after cessation of therapy, so that treatment must be continued indefinitely to maintain protection against fracture. Enthusiasm for prolonged hormone replacement therapy is falling in the light of increasing public awareness of breast cancer risk, and weakening of the evidence for cardioprotective benefits. The selective oestrogen receptor modulators, already in use for oestrogen-sensitive breast tumours, have recently been evaluated as a treatment for osteoporosis. One of these, raloxifene, has been shown to reduce the rate of vertebral fractures in postmenopausal women with osteoporosis, but an effect on non-vertebral fractures has not been demonstrated. While oestrogen-receptor positive breast cancer incidence is significantly reduced during up to 4 years of therapy, it is unclear what effect cessation of treatment may have on incidence (i.e. if a tumour is suppressed rather than prevented, breast cancer incidence will rise on cessation of selective oestrogen replacement modulator therapy). Raloxifene does not stimulate the endometrium and thus its use is not associated with withdrawal bleeding. It does not alleviate and may exacerbate vasomotor symptoms associated with the menopause and is therefore not suitable for use in perimenopausal women with active menopausal symptoms. As with conventional hormone replacement therapy, there is a two- to three-fold increase in the relative risk of venous thromboembolism. The effects of raloxifene on cardiovascular disease and cognitive function have not been established. Several large randomised controlled trials are now ongoing which should, in the next decade, elucidate the effects both of HRT and of raloxifene on these important end points.

Bisphosphonates

Alendronate and risedronate have both been shown to reduce fracture incidence by approximately 50%, both at vertebral and non-vertebral sites in postmenopausal women with osteoporosis, and are also indicated for the prevention and treatment of corticosteroid induced osteoporosis. However, their cost-effectiveness may be limited in women without prevalent fracture. Nonetheless, developments in this group of drugs (which also have other indications) continue, with an emphasis upon:

- onset time to fracture prevention (alendronate and risedronate reduce fracture risk within 12–18 months)

- improved gastrointestinal tolerability (therefore better safety and compliance)
- reduced dose frequency – there is some evidence that efficacy is determined by accumulated dose rather than dose frequency; therefore, once weekly or less frequent doses may reduce adverse effects and improve compliance (though it is not clear that infrequent doses are taken any more reliably than daily treatment), while retaining beneficial skeletal effects
- bolus intravenous agents will particularly suit such induction–maintenance regimens.

Although bisphosphonates have a long skeletal half-life, a drug which has been incorporated into bone is not bioavailable and there is increasing evidence that bone loss may resume after the cessation of bisphosphonate therapy. In the case of the most potent bisphosphonates, marked suppression of bone turnover is associated with increased mineralisation of bone which may, at least in theory, lead to adverse effects on bone strength. Thus a prolonged effect on the skeleton may not be desirable.

A recent trial with alendronate showed significant increases in bone mineral density and reduced vertebral fracture risk in men with osteoporosis and it is likely that bisphosphonates will be increasingly used for this indication in the future.

Calcium and vitamin D

A calcium intake of at least 1 g/day, with or without supplementation, is recommended by the World Health Organization taskforce among others. Though an essential physiological requirement from birth (and indeed *in utero*), the role of calcium both in the pathogenesis and the management of osteoporosis is controversial. There is evidence that supplementation in childhood is associated with significant increases in bone mineral density, raising the possibility that this approach might be used as a public health measure to increase bone mineral density in the population. However, there is no evidence that such intervention would reduce fractures later in life. Calcium supplementation has also been shown to have beneficial effects on bone mineral density in premenopausal, perimenopausal and postmenopausal women. However, evidence for a reduction in fracture rate in the latter group is inconsistent and calcium should be regarded as an adjunct to therapy in those with low dietary calcium intake rather than as a definitive treatment.

Photosynthesis of vitamin D provides adequate levels in most age groups, although vitamin D deficiency or insufficiency is common in many elderly populations and, as a result of secondary hyperparathyroidism, has adverse effects on bone health. Vitamin D_3 (800 iu) with calcium (500 mg to 1.2 g) has been shown to reduce non-vertebral and hip fracture rates in elderly populations, although whether vitamin D alone is sufficient to produce this benefit is currently unknown. The active metabolite of vitamin D_3, 1,25 dihydroxyvitamin D_3, (calcitriol) has been shown to have beneficial effects on bone mineral density in postmenopausal women with osteoporosis, although the fracture prevention data are inconsistent. The place of calcitriol, or its synthetic analogue 1α-calcidol, in the management of osteoporosis thus remains unclear.

Calcitonin

Calcitonin may be administered as an intranasal spray or subcutaneous injection. Although beneficial effects on spinal bone mineral density have been demonstrated in several studies, its antifracture efficacy is less well established.

Future antiresorptive agents

There are numerous potential targets for reducing bone resorption. Examples include the following:

- inhibitors of integrin binding and of the H^+-ATPase required for demineralisation
- inhibitors of cathepsin K (an osteoclast specific enzyme which degrades bone matrix)
- analogues of endogenous osteoprotegerin, a soluble receptor which inhibits osteoclast formation.

The next generation of osteoporosis treatment – anabolic agents

"Bone building" drugs have been sought for decades, a reminder that the journey from hypothetical concept to bench to bedside is frequently long and tortuous. Increased understanding of the capacity of bone to repair micro- and macro-trauma, together with advances in pharmaceutical development, offers the potential for rational design of agents with the potential for significant improvements in the management of osteoporosis.

Parathyroid hormone and its analogues

Under normal circumstances, endogenous pulses of parathyroid hormone stimulate bone resorption to maintain serum calcium levels. However, when administered as intermittent (subcutaneous) injections, parathyroid hormone increases bone mass both by stimulating *de novo* bone formation and by the combination of increased activation frequency and positive remodelling balance. The 1–34 amino terminal portion of the hormone (similar to parathyroid related peptide) is synthetically produced (recombinant technology) and its effects have been studied in patients with osteoporosis. A recent study in postmenopausal women with established osteoporosis showed a 65% reduction in vertebral fractures, and a 54% reduction in non-vertebral fractures at a dose of 20 µg daily for 1–2 years with side-effects comparable to placebo. As accelerated bone less may follow withdrawal of PTH, it is likely that anti-resorptive therapy will be used following PTH treatment.

Although the requirement for parenteral administration may reduce tolerability and compliance, methods for its delivery and that of many peptides, particularly insulin, are likely to improve considerably in the coming decade or so.

Strontium

First investigated over 30 years ago, strontium in low doses with calcium increased osteoid (new, not yet mineralised bone), increased cancellous bone volume and increased bone strength in animal studies. However, high doses reduce the production of endogenous calcitriol and impair mineralisation. The drug, therefore, may have a relatively narrow therapeutic window. Nonetheless, significant increases in spine bone mineral density have been demonstrated in one human study where the drug was well tolerated and Phase III clinical trials are ongoing.

Statins

Some observational studies have reported higher bone mineral density and reduced fracture incidence in postmenopausal women on statin therapy, although this finding has not been universal. Recent technological developments have enabled screening of a wide range of natural and other agents for their osteogenic potential, one mechanism being through increased expression of the promoter for bone morphogenic protein (BMP) 2. Some of the statins, particularly cirivastatin and atorvastatin, are potent agents in this assay. There are interesting parallels between the proposed mechanism of action of statins and of nitrogen containing bisphosphonates, as both act on the mevalonate pathway of cholesterol biosynthesis, although statins appear to exert their effect mainly on osteoblasts whereas the bisphosphonates act primarily on the osteoclast. The currently available statins are specifically designed to target the liver but there is now considerable interest in the development of statins which target the bone.

Growth factors

Growth factors produced by the osteoblast include transforming growth factor beta (*TGF-β*), IGF (insulin-like growth factor)-1 and -2, and BMP-2 and -7. These have a number of potential applications, including fracture repair, corrective procedures, management of bone loss following trauma or tumour excision, and osteoporosis. The following observations are relevant to these:

- Injection of BMP into the body of a fractured vertebra has been shown to increase vertebral height, bone density and strength.
- *TGF-β*, IGF-1 and BMP-7 (also known as osteogenic protein 1) induce osteoblast activity in cell cultures; however, it may take a decade to translate this into an effective therapy. Gene therapy may be developed relatively quickly as a way of delivering these factors to fracture sites or perhaps to other areas which may be vulnerable (e.g. in the hemiparetic hip).
- Transcription factors of the growth factor BMP-2 are deactivated by a proteosome, inhibitors of which are available and have been used in laboratory models with promising results.

Another development from the orthopaedic literature is the injection of polymethacrylate bone cement into recently fractured vertebrae, with improved mechanical strength, increased vertebral height and reduced pain. However, studies to date are small, and an increased risk of fracture in the adjacent vertebrae causes concern. Nonetheless, this is a development that will be followed with interest.

Other developments in intervention

As stated in the WHO constitution, the cooperation of an educated public is essential to achieve global health for all. Better informing the public about osteoporosis risk (improving case finding) and about relevant lifestyle factors will be an important future target. While the impact of any lifestyle intervention is likely to be quite small for any one individual, the potential for "shifting to the right" the normal curve of bone mineral density could be significant. Although a great deal of the activity in this area is likely to come from voluntary organisations, the physician's role as educator will expand as public expectations for accurate information and guidance from the medical community increases.

Monitoring therapy

There is some disagreement at present over how best to monitor the efficacy of interventions for osteoporosis and, indeed, whether this should be done at all. On the one hand, the majority of apparent non-responders are non-compliant or pursue a lifestyle which renders therapy ineffective and, since the number of true non-responders to the more efficacious treatments is low, it is arguable whether there is any role for monitoring of therapy (consistent with the principles of screening). On the other hand, it may be difficult to persuade patients to take long term therapy that does not result in symptomatic improvement and may cause side-effects, without some means of reassurance that the treatment is having the desired effect.

There also remain unanswered questions regarding the period which should elapse before seeking a response to treatment, and conversely how soon a person should be considered a non-responder. Bone mineral density is the gold standard surrogate marker of fracture risk – how satisfactory is it in monitoring response to therapy? What alternatives are there? Also what impact will such information have on management (i.e. what is the cost effectiveness of any such monitoring)?

The rate of change in bone mineral density is greatest in the spine, and this site is therefore preferred for monitoring. The precision error of spine measurements is about 1%; a reliably detectable difference (2.8 times the coefficient of variance) must therefore be around 3%, which would usually require at least two years of treatment. At the hip, where rates of change in bone mineral density are less, it may take three or more years before the response to treatment can be assessed. Changes occurring in individuals over relatively short periods of time are difficult to interpret because of the imprecision of measurements and the phenomenon of regression to the mean.

Reflecting rates of bone turnover, biochemical markers change more quickly than bone mineral density. Within six months, reductions in resorption and formation markers have been noted; the degree of difference means that a statistically significant change is more readily identified. However, the correlation of these changes in turnover markers in an individual patient with increased bone mineral density, and more importantly with reduction of fracture rates, has yet to be established.

If non-responders are identified early, there must be a hierarchy of treatment to identify "more potent" strategies to protect these patients. While some alternatives, particularly combinations of currently available therapies, will be investigated in the next few years, it remains to be seen whether those who do not respond to one strategy are likely to respond to an alternative – if not, the value of drug monitoring will certainly be challenged.

Future delivery of osteoporosis care

As in many disciplines, osteoporosis diagnosis and management will move to primary care and will be increasingly driven by protocols, algorithms and guidelines from international and local bodies, experts focussing instead on research, appraisal of new data and ensuring that guidelines continue to offer effective management.

In the UK resources in the primary care setting are already increasing with the development of primary care trusts. Financial incentives for cost efficiency are increasingly dominant and elements of private care are returning. Options that an individual patient may believe to be worth the cost (akin to decisions about purchasing insurance) may not be cost effective for society (where cost to prevent one fracture is the dominant argument). This can easily be envisaged as applying to routine postmenopausal or treatment monitoring dual energy x ray absorptiometry, or to specific treatments (for example, anabolic therapies or even bisphosphonates).

Worldwide, similar debates apply to all models of healthcare delivery. Where state-supported insurance schemes are in place, the underwriters may take an active role in requiring early detection and primary prevention, or may limit cover to those with established osteoporosis (already in place in much of Europe). An unacceptable burden of cost in caring for the elderly is predicted to fall on a diminishing young population. This has prompted proposals, including Tribunals for Maintenance of Parents (Singapore) where the elderly will have legal recourse to obtain a minimum standard of care from their relatives, or contributory insurance schemes to cover health care after 75 years of age (Europe). Despite the recent move by the pharmaceutical industry to provide antiretroviral therapy to the developing world to combat HIV/AIDS, it is highly unlikely that such philanthropic gestures will include osteoporosis. Therefore, the ageing population of South East Asia and South America, where up to 75% of hip fractures are predicted to occur over the next 30 years, is unlikely to benefit from the advances so eagerly anticipated here. The equitable reallocation of global resources to the world's people is a discussion that extends far beyond any vision of osteoporosis.

A vision of the future – a community in 2030?

- Zara, aged one, has her compulsory "SMALL" (screening for major ailments in later life) at the NHS primary care centre. Family history, physical measurements and a genome analysis are input to an artificial neural network that calculates a risk profile, becoming part of a central record and embedded in her personal swipe card. She may have no osteoporotic predisposition, may risk a suboptimal peak bone mass or be a fast loser, or may have increased vitamin D, calcium or other requirement earning a bonus on her child health allowance to obtain the required supplement. Throughout her schooling, she will receive health education, regular exercise, 500 mg calcium supplement and a fruit supplement.
- Brittney, Zara's 12 year old sister has her growth rate assessed at a school clinic. If in the lowest quartile, or if she is at risk of a low peak bone mass, she receives anabolic therapy throughout the pubertal growth phase.
- Zara and Brittney's mother, Sarah, 35, is a smoker, exercises little, and an ultrasound at the supermarket shows her to be at risk of osteoporosis. Lifestyle modification is advised; if treatment is required, only 50% of the cost is borne by health insurance (because her risk factors are self-inflicted, her swipe card indicating no genetic or family risk).
- Aunt Beth attends a compulsory well woman perimenopausal review, which includes ultrasound and bone turnover marker profile; together with the "high risk" profile on her swipe card, a coupon is issued for the private dual energy x ray absorptiometry facility. She joins others having self-funded dual energy x ray

absorptiometry (outside the National Health recommendations). Her genetic, physiological (turnover marker) and bone typing (density and stiffness index) are combined to issue the relevant section of the "GROT" (global recommendations for osteoporosis treatment)", which obtains free medication. (If the GROT from self-funded dual energy x ray absorptiometry recommends treatment, the scan cost is reimbursed.)

- Non-protocol medications, including the bisphosphonates for those without fracture or other risk, may be obtained at full cost to the client.

- Bone turnover is rechecked after six months, and one year of depot parathyroid analogue prescribed if increases in formation markers are suboptimal. If resorption markers fail to fall substantially, combination antiresorptive therapy is used (bisphosphonates given three monthly as intravenous bolus injections until sustained reduction is obtained, and in response to turnover markers thereafter).

- If hormone replacement therapy or a selective oestrogen replacement modulator is prescribed for other indications (e.g. cancer prevention programme), dual energy x ray absorptiometry is not done, but turnover is assessed as for other clients.

- NHS retirement screening (at age 70) offers measurement of hip dual energy x ray absorptiometry and biochemical markers of bone turnover, those with normal bone density and a normal rate of loss being reviewed 5 yearly. Those whose risk profile (T-score of -2.5, or prevalent fracture) indicates treatment will receive bolus intravenous bisphosphonate therapy. If formation markers are below the reference range or a further fracture occurs, anabolic therapy (parathyroid hormone or an osteospecific statin) will be prescribed.

- Those who sustain osteoporotic fractures who failed to attend screening will be liable for the short term costs entailed.

While some of these strategies are perhaps Orwellian, and some of the therapeutic interventions somewhat speculative, the scenario highlights the direction future developments might take. The ideal will surely be met when any name from any part of the world may be substituted, the programme perhaps supported by globally funded health care through the World Health Organization or similar bodies, and when people can continue to live a full and active life until their still inevitable death.

Reference

1 Writing Group of the Bone and Tooth Society of Great Britain and the Royal College of Physicians. *Osteoporosis. Clinical guidelines for prevention and treatment. Update on pharmacological interventions and an algorithm for management*. London: Royal College of Physicians, 2000.

Recommended reading

Adachi JD, Olszynski WP, Hanley DA *et al*. Management of corticosteroid induced osteoporosis. *Semin Arthritis Rheum* 2000;**29**:228–51.

Boden SD. Bioactive factors for bone tissue engineering. *Clin Orthop* 1999;**367**(suppl):s84–s98.

Compston J, Ralston S, eds. *Osteoporosis and Bone Biology: the state of the art*. London: International Medical Press, 2000.

Cosman F, Lindsay R. Is PTH a therapeutic option for osteoporosis? A review of the clinical evidence. *Calcif Tiss Int* 1998;**62**:475–80.

Cummings SR, Palermo L, Browner W *et al*. for the Fracture Intervention Trial Research Group. Monitoring of treatment with bone densitometry: misleading changes and regression towards the mean. *JAMA* 2000; **283**:1318–21.

Eastell R, Boyle IT, Compston J *et al*. Management of male osteoporosis: report of the UK consensus group. *Q J Med* 1998;**91**:71–92.

Eisman JA. The genetics of osteoporosis. *Endocrinol Rev* 1999;**20**:788–804.

Genant HK, Cooper C, Poor G *et al*. Interim report and recommendations of the WHO Task Force for Osteoporosis. *Osteoporosis Int* 2000;**10**:259–64.

Gluer CC. Quantitative ultrasound techniques for the assessment of osteoporosis. *J Bone Min Res* 1997;**12**:1280–8.

Kanis JA, Gluer CC for the Committee of Scientific Advisors, International Osteoporosis Foundation. An update on the diagnosis and assessment of osteoporosis with densitometry. *Osteoporosis Int* 2000;**11**:192–202.

Levis S, Altman R. Bone densitometry: clinical considerations. *Arthritis Rheum* 1998;**41**:577–87.

Manolagas SC. Birth and death of bone cells: basic regulatory mechanisms and implications for the pathogenesis and treatment of osteoporosis. *Endocrinol Rev* 2000;**21**:115–37.

Mundy G *et al*. Stimulation of bone formation *in vitro* and in rodents by statins. *Science* 1999;**286**:1946–9.

Reginster JY. Promising new agents in osteoporosis. *Drugs Res Dev* 1999;**1**:195–201.

Seibel MJ, Woitge H. Basic principles and clinical applications of biochemical markers of bone metabolism. *J Clin Densitometry* 1999;**2**:299–321.

Von Mühlen D, Visby-Lunde A, Barrett-Connor E, Bettencourt R. Evaluation of SCORE in older caucasian women. *Osteoporosis Int* 1999;**10**:79–84.

Writing Group of the Bone and Tooth Society of Great Britain and the Royal College of Physicians. *Osteoporosis. Clinical guidelines for prevention and treatment. Update on pharmacological interventions and an algorithm for management*. London: Royal College of Physicians, 2000.

7: The future diagnosis and management of chronic musculoskeletal pain

PETER CROFT

Chronic musculoskeletal pain affects between one in three and one in six of the adult population in Western countries. Osteoarthritis is the dominant problem in the elderly; in younger adults, low back pain, neck and upper limb pain, and chronic widespread pain occupy centre-stage. In many countries, these conditions are the leading cause of disability and of working days lost, and are one of the two or three most frequent reasons for seeking health care. Chronic musculoskeletal pain is prevalent throughout the world, but the frequency of seeking health care and the impact on systems of health and social care varies dramatically. This is partly a demographic issue – the greater the life expectancy, the proportionately higher proportion of the population will have such non-fatal problems – but is also related to cultural and social characteristics of different populations.

Understanding chronic musculoskeletal pain

I want to start by making a distinction between progress in "understanding" pain and likely developments in the practical "application" of new knowledge. There is a common assumption that the former will inevitably lead to the latter. This is a misconception. A study might estimate the likely contribution of inheritance to spinal disc degeneration; the press release then gives a strong hint that this research will lead to cures for low back pain. The study is well performed and advances our understanding of spinal disc degeneration. However, other studies have established that most low back pain is unrelated to spinal disc disease, and knowing that disc disease is mostly an inherited genetic problem does not mean that it can be or should be "reversed" or "treated" – a general problem for genetic studies at the current state of our knowledge – nor does it mean that this knowledge will have any relevance or applicability to the problem of chronic back pain.

However, the last decades of the old millennium did bring clear advances in the science of pain. These are important in their own right but they also have profound implications for how we will conceive and understand chronic musculoskeletal pain in the future, regardless of whether or not they have obvious therapeutic applications. A brief summary is needed, with apologies to experts in the field for the crudeness of my exposition.[1-3]

The old idea was that a source of injury produces signals to the brain which are interpreted as pain. The pain sensation can be blocked by analgesic drugs, but the cure for the pain depends on healing the damaged tissue. The new idea is that our nervous system is more dynamic and adaptable than this, and that it can change in response to pain stimuli in ways which can persist even when the source of pain has been removed and the site of injury repaired. This "plasticity" of the nervous system is affected by all sorts of influences – other pains for example or higher brain functions such as emotions and psychological states – and in turn can affect other parts of the nervous system, even the motor functions. This provides a biological explanation for the finding that pain can persist in the absence of continuing local damage and under the influence of, for example, anxiety. The original source of pain can disappear, and the pain continues as an active memory within the nervous system.

This is the crucial, albeit over-simplified, picture of pain with which we enter the twenty-first century. There will be future refinements to this model, notably in the much broader field of understanding consciousness, but already it is clear that what follows from this development in neuroscience is going to shape our approach to and management of chronic musculoskeletal disease in the next decades. Much of this chapter is concerned with this.

Will the medical perspective on chronic musculoskeletal pain change?

The importance of traditional diagnosis will decline

The first major implication of the new ideas is that they provide support for clinicians to advance out of their nineteenth-century view of diagnosis, which is still concerned primarily with seeking a local pathology for chronic pain and making a diagnosis at the site of the pain as the end-point of their deliberations. That is not to say that identifying the small minority of patients with serious underlying problems such as tumours or infections is not important, but that for back pain, neck and upper limb pain, and widespread pain, there is no evidence that searching for a local diagnosis carries much benefit for the patient.

Traditional clinicopathological diagnostic medicine is likely to die out as a mainstream version of pain management. Effective "red flag" spotting will be the clinical order of the day, in which the frontline purpose of diagnosis is to identify serious pathologies for which we have specific treatments.

There is evidence to support such a change of direction, for example the demonstration that spinal osteoarthritis on x ray is a poor guide to the presence of back pain. However, the objection to the old system of diagnosing chronic musculoskeletal pain in terms of local pathology is less that it is intellectually often without foundation, rather that there is no evidence that it gives rise to effective treatment. Indeed it may encourage wrong approaches to treatment by patient and clinician alike.[4]

Further support for a change of direction comes from the neurobiological studies which have provided us with a reason for seeing that pain is about the higher cerebral functions and their relationship to the outside world as much as it is about local injury – important as the latter might be in the initiation and localisation of pain. As one observer has put it, "Back pain is more than pain in the back".[5]

My belief that this change of direction will actually occur is based on the observation that things are already changing in that direction. Low back pain management guidelines point out that most patients cannot be diagnosed, and that triage is the key step – identify the important "red flags", diagnose the conditions that can be managed (notably sciatic nerve compression), and then consider the rest (i.e. the majority) as a problem of pain and disability and not as a challenge to pathological know-how.

Imaging will improve

The baby must not be thrown out with the bathwater however – the capacity to diagnose local pathologies will improve; the science of imaging is likely to get better. However, there is no evidence that improving our view of the minutiae of structural abnormalities in joint and bone, in the absence of clear clinical pointers to diagnosis, will serve the cause of most patients with chronic pain particularly well. There are two exceptions to this.

Firstly, diagnosis of acute musculoskeletal pain. This is relevant because early treatment of acute musculoskeletal injury is one means to prevent chronic pain. The more efficient and effective the diagnosis and management of injury, the better the prognosis might be – although this needs to be researched.[6]

Secondly, improved accuracy and technique in local diagnosis may progress clinical management of "red flags". If a diagnosis of cancer or infection or inflammation is a critical first step in managing musculoskeletal pain, then improved diagnostic techniques will help, but only in the context of clinical selection. Efficient use of x rays in back pain, for example, depends on their use being made subordinate to clinical indications and not on being a screening instrument for all pain. Newer imaging methods, such as magnetic resonance techniques, may improve the accuracy of diagnosis in selected patients, but currently will not substitute for symptoms and signs in an extensive way, given the sheer number of patients who present to health care with musculoskeletal pain. Cheapness, accuracy and safety of new techniques together may conspire to change this however. Although doctors fondly imagine that their clinical consultation with the patient remains the best initial guide to the presence of "red flag" problems, it is sentiment alone to argue that machines will never replace this activity.

Alternatives for classifying chronic musculoskeletal pain

1. Categorise pain severity and the disability it causes

Progress in classification of chronic musculoskeletal pain needs to go in a direction opposite to that of increasing the accuracy of local tissue imaging. The evidence suggests that many syndromes of chronic regional pain, although initially dictated by local injury as to their location, are very similar to each other once persistence is established. Common influences on chronicity, similar effects of different chronic pain syndromes on peoples' lives, and the importance of pain management compared with attempts at curing local pathology, all suggest that clinical classification of chronic musculoskeletal pain will be more about pain severity and the presence of factors which predict or maintain chronicity than about distinguishing different chronic musculoskeletal pain syndromes. Such classification will be equally concerned with non-specific influences on pain persistence – previous experience of pain, psychological factors, socioeconomic pressures – as it is with clinical or diagnostic characteristics.

The current evidence from case series and epidemiology is that these non-specific influences are the strongest prognostic factors in chronic musculoskeletal pain. However, it cannot be assumed that tackling these factors will itself be useful and effective in treating and preventing chronic pain. Evidence for this has yet to be gathered – trials of interventions are likely to dominate research in this field for some years to come. Current guidelines for managing low back pain are, however, reflecting the view that maintaining activity, dealing with the psychology of pain, and accepting that adaptation rather than cure is the target, may be the most effective approaches to the management of chronic pain – along with good pain relief and appropriate physical treatments.[7]

2. Classify the underlying mechanisms of pain persistence

The shift to an acceptance that pain is important in itself rather than simply as a pointer to the "diagnosis" lays open the possibility that we can apply the findings of pain physiology in a practical way. Various authors have proposed a clinical classification of chronic pain in terms of neurobiology and broad control mechanisms of pain in the body (for example Woolf[8]). The processing of pain by the nervous system would become the focus of clinical concern and such a classification would directly reflect the new ideas from neurobiology and could lead to its own diagnostic lexicon.

However, we should be cautious about this proposal: the usefulness to the patient in pain of such a mechanism based classification would need to be proven and justified. The argument goes that such knowledge and classification will open a whole world of targeted treatments for pain relief and prevention of chronicity.

An alternative prediction (which I favour) is that such classifications will be more useful to the understanding of chronic musculoskeletal pain than to its practical management. This will be proven wrong if there is a therapeutic breakthrough based on pain mechanisms and on diagnosing a specific abnormality of the pain pathway that can be corrected.

The problem of chronic pain without an obvious underlying cause

There are likely to be further advances, triggered by the new neurobiology, in our understanding of patients with chronic musculoskeletal pain. In particular there must be a reason why plasticity and pain memory kick into action in some people but not others. For some patients, their personal history seems a living embodiment of how physical injury and psychological influences might combine over many years to produce a chronic pain syndrome resistant to easy treatment, such as the woman with fibromyalgia who has suffered years of physical battering at the hands of an abusive husband. But for many others, even if there are such environmental triggers, the explanation of their proneness to amplify and to develop pain dissociated from local injury or pathology still needs to be found.

My prediction is that a science of this will develop which will explain it in terms of neurobiology and human physiology. We do not need to assume that this will give us the key to simple therapy, given the likely complexities of the cultural and social and psychological background to it all. It might turn out to have a genetic component, or to depend on early influences on fetal or infant development. Pain amplification in particular will gain a hypothesis and theory as to why some people develop it and not others – more probably from developmental biology than from genetics. It is likely that, as Loeser and Melzack summarise,[2] the mechanisms for environmental influences on central processing of pain, the role of injury-induced stress in influencing chronic pain development, and the role of emotion and cognition (and, as Wall has pointed out, expectations) will be clarified in the next 10–20 years, and we will have models of how the chronic pain experience develops.

From a clinical point of view, this will shed particular light on those patients who represent the majority of sufferers with chronic musculoskeletal pain and whose pain we still do not understand. The main examples are sufferers with back pain and chronic widespread pain. Such chronic pain syndromes are common, and represent an increasing burden on the welfare and medicolegal systems. In the new century the challenge is clear – to understand and help people with a severe core pain, which may affect different parts of the body to a varying extent, and which is resistant to many therapies. The future may bring an insight to why these patients are different and how we can prevent their problem developing in the first place. Why should injury or "everyday" somatisation of distress and anxiety as pain become for some people a long term and crippling burden?

Future developments in understanding and explaining chronic pain will have a broader remit. Not only will these ideas unify our approach to chronic pain syndromes so that they appear more alike than different, but other syndromes will also be understood within the same models. There is strong evidence for overlap between chronic pain and other syndromes, such as chronic fatigue or irritable bowel, for which a clear peripheral pathology does not exist. The biology of somatisation is likely to embrace a wide range of chronic symptoms.

In summary

A patient's pain will be treated at face value and will be assessed on the basis of its impact on people's lives and the social and psychological context in which it occurs, and perhaps on the basis of the neurophysiological mechanism for the pain, but not on a chase for local pathology. The exception will be where the pain is clearly best managed by attention to peripheral damage – for example, osteoarthritis of the knee treated by knee joint replacement. The nineteenth-century approach, based on the constant hunt for local pathology, has ended up with most chronic pain being a failure of pain treatment.[9] The new ideas, biologically based, place the emphasis on the pain and the patient with the pain.

Will drug treatments change?

The rhetoric is persuasive: staggering advances in our understanding of the biological basis for pain will continue until the map is complete. Patients will have their pain classified in terms of the specific part of the neural map which is responsible, and pharmacology will attempt to target new therapies at those specific points.

History, however, does not provide encouragement for supposing that specific chemical treatments will develop on the back of more precise knowledge. The problem of extrapolating from the science of understanding to its practical application is what one French historian of pain has observed as the discontinuity in the rate of discoveries of advances in pain treatments – centuries of no advance or even regression, but then "the rhythm of new discoveries became suddenly accelerated".[10]

This might be because all medical advances occur by accident rather than being driven neatly by the application of the latest advance in scientific understanding. By contrast, one leading pain scientist has a more generous view when recalling the period of accelerated pharmaceutical advances in the early twentieth century. However, of the past 50 years, he summarises "only two advances have appeared in the treatment of pain from the major drug companies ... and they are both coincidental side-effects: some antiepileptic drugs are effective in neuropathic pain, and some antidepressant drugs are usefully analgesic".[1]

Musculoskeletal pain offers a prime example of the old model of chronic pain. Continuing stimulation from an area of tissue damage, which provides input to the central area of pain perception, is one possible model of osteoarthritis of the hip and knee. For patients with advanced radiographic evidence of osteoarthritis in these joints, the next decades are likely to see continuing success in relieving pain and restoring mobility by surgical replacement of joints and removal of the peripheral stimulus to pain. However, such patients represent a minority of all older people with joint pain who form the group with "clinical osteoarthritis". Many others in this group actually fit more closely with a model of chronic pain – more obviously represented by back problems or fibromyalgia – in which pain has become dislocated from the site of peripheral damage, and for whom changes in pain processing are the key to understanding their continuing pain. Treatments such as surgery are unlikely to provide relief in such cases[11]; nor are single modalities of treatment which address only one component of the pain experience likely to fare any better.

Against this background, we have to interpret the hopes of those who are concluding their summaries of the huge advances in our understanding of pain mechanisms by claims for what this will mean in terms of pharmacological advance. As an example[8]: "We are poised to move from a treatment paradigm that has been almost entirely empirical to one that will be derived from an understanding of the actual mechanisms involved in the pathogenesis of pain". Well, just possibly – and beta-blockers and the H_2 antagonists offer analogies that pharmacological advances can occur in this way. However, within the musculoskeletal field, decades of brilliant unravelling of the inflammatory response has not given us a magic bullet.

The shallowness of current claims is highlighted by phrases about the new class of non-steroidal anti-inflammatory drugs known as COX-2 inhibitors, which state that they have "generated excitement". Yet this class of drugs is offering no added efficacy for pain – it is simply targeting the inflammatory response more specifically and leaving the lining of the digestive system alone. In other words the advance lies in the possibility of reducing some iatrogenic side effects. The roles of the pharmaceutical industry and the commercial imperative in driving the therapeutic evangelism that surrounds the genuinely exciting advances of pain physiology and pain genetics need to be highlighted.

For pain poses a conundrum for pharmacological advance. The biomedical scientists have provided us with a clear rationale and mechanisms for why culture, society, affect and cognition, fears and expectations, have such a profound and important influence on the chronicity of pain. And yet some of these same scientists would have us believe that the true virtue of their unveiling of the mechanisms of pain is that we have an array of specific chemical targets for newly fashioned therapies. An equal argument would be that if we can identify anything that alters affect and cognition and beliefs in the right direction – a homoeopathic physician who, say, spends an hour with a patient alleviating fears, creating expectations in an atmosphere of trust, reducing anxiety, addressing domestic topics – then why not bet on that? Indeed there may be less uncertainty in that, since it is all very well to target a piece of the mechanism, but history tells us that upsetting the homeostasis and equilibrium of body systems can have bad as well as good effects. The COX-2 story provides a good example of this, with one of the experts on this class of drugs pointing out that inhibiting COX-2 activity may paradoxically promote some types of inflammatory activity.[12]

It would be foolish to make this gaze into the crystal ball of the pharmacological future at the beginning of the twenty-first century exclusively Luddite, given the fantastic rate of technological change over the last 50 years. Brand new agents to treat musculoskeletal pain and nip chronicity in the bud might appear in a side effect-free nirvana of applied pharmacology. But it would be equally foolish to assume that the amazing advances in understanding, imaging and integrating the pain story – which I do believe will be unravelled in all its complexity in the coming decades – will automatically result in great new analgesic drugs. Indeed there are some reasons to suppose that, for pain particularly, the pharmaceutical path, good as it is, should not be seen as the only way in which pain management can advance.

In summary, I think it unlikely that new targeted therapies in chronic musculoskeletal pain will produce major advances in management, but I would be happy to be proven wrong.

Milder grounds for optimism lie in the continuing advance of opioid science and the refinement of its application.[13] The safe and effective deployment of opioids has been one of the major breakthroughs of humane pain therapy, although internationally it remains unevenly applied, and the role of these drugs in the management of chronic musculoskeletal pain is certainly not clear. Advances in multiple therapies that harness the endogenous system and reduce the side effects of opioids will allow experiments to address their possible role in chronic musculoskeletal pain. Cannibinoids are another traditional drug group which may have a similarly enhanced role in coming years.

What will be the role of the placebo in pain management?

My prediction is that there will be many impeccably carried out randomised controlled trials of pain management using complementary therapies, and that they will universally show an overall positive effect which is only a little higher than placebo. The role of expectation and the power of the placebo is becoming a challenge to our capacity to harness and use the placebo effect therapeutically. We have emerged from the end of the twentieth century with strong experiments to show that what may be the most important thing in placebo controlled trials of pain treatments is neither the randomisation, nor the efficacy of the active drug, but the amazingly powerful effect on pain of the placebo itself. Coupled with these is convincing biological science to explain just why suggestion and expectation and fear reduction might be such positive influences in reducing pain.[14] This leads me to suppose that the science of the non-specific effects of care and treatment will be the focus of a whole tranche of pain research and that ways of harnessing these (or the parts of existing therapies which harness them already) will come to be seen as the cornerstone of both mainstream and complementary pain therapy science rather than the study of the little bit of extra efficacy that might come from the real thing as compared with the sham thing. Therapies will not lose respectability because they are little different from placebo, but they may gain respectability from the demonstrable power of their non-specific effect, and perhaps from their lack of side effects, compared with magic bullets from the pharmaceutical industry.

But there is a paradox, one that Richard Asher knew and wrote about 40 years ago[15]: "It is better to prescribe something that is useless, but which you and the patient both believe in, than to admit that you do not know what to do." The crisis for placebo and expectation research is that, once you have shown rationally that it does not matter too much what you do as long as the patients like it, believe in it and expects it to make them better, how can you promote the irrational as rationally the most effective measure to reduce pain? How can you support something in the knowledge that it is only the belief and not the substance which is effective?

One of the optimistic things about all this relates to the fact that the opinions and prophecies of experts who stand at opposite sides of the biological–cultural divide are couched in the same language. This suggests that a major potential advance in chronic pain management in the forthcoming decades will be an ability to talk about the social and cultural in biological terms whilst avoiding solutions which reduce to the exclusively biochemical. Patrick Wall for instance, one of the outstanding figures in biological pain science in the twentieth century, stated: "A crucial component is the patient's belief that it works – for the patient who benefits, it matters not a toss why it works". Arthur Kleinman, one of the great figures in anthropological pain research, quotes a physician, Spiro, suggesting that "the placebo effect – the non-specific therapeutic effect of the doctor–patient relationship – although it is despised in medical research because it confounds a clear-cut understanding of the specificity of successful treatments – is in fact the essence of effective clinical care".[16]

So future decades should see the scientific gaze turn on the proportion of clinical effectiveness which is about the non-specifics of dealing with pain and suffering rather than be myopically and exclusively concerned with the usually smaller proportion of effectiveness which might be attributed to the particular chemical molecule being tested. And let it do so with a neurobiological model of how it might work, a model which actually asks whether single chemical approaches to the problem of chronic musculoskeletal pain are doomed to failure if taken out of the clinical, social and psychological context of the patient suffering from pain.

What will be the role of non-pharmacological pain management?

Strong evidence now exists that the psychological status of the individual – emotions and beliefs, attitudes and learned behaviour – as well as the social, cultural and economic circumstances in which they live, are crucial influences on why people develop chronic and persisting musculoskeletal pain. The biology of pain presents us with an explanation of the neurological mechanisms as to why this is so. The question now to be addressed is the extent to which therapies and interventions directed at beliefs, attitudes, behaviour and circumstances may be effective. Here there is currently conflict of opinion.[1]

The disagreement seems to be about the extent to which chronic pain should be ascribed to psychological status and how far psychological approaches should dominate treatment strategies. This is partly again an issue of language and attitude. Psychological approaches tend to be interpreted as somehow denying the reality of pain or the possibility of pain relief. There are objections also to the rather punitive notion of rehabilitation and return to work when they are employed as sticks rather than carrots in chronic pain management programmes. However, physical approaches to chronic musculoskeletal pain have clearly failed to help or prevent most problems, and psychological therapies, orientated towards behaviours and beliefs, are concerned to take people seriously and to help them cope, and in neurophysiological terms to alter higher cortical influences on pain persistence and perception. Differences arise because effects rather than causes of pain seem to be the focus of pain management programmes. Yet this fits with the notion of chronic pain as a symptom dislocated from its primary cause and whose persistence is irrevocably tied up with the effects it has.

In terms of the future, it seems unlikely that there will be major advances in techniques of psychological treatment or principles of pain management. However, there are ways in which things might be improved. As a strategy, cognitive behavioural therapy and multidisciplinary pain management are time consuming and, given the prevalence of chronic pain, it is inappropriate to see them as widely available treatments. However, selection and targeting of patients could be improved so that the psychologists and therapists are not simply presented with far advanced syndromes to unravel. More controversially, there is the need to develop brief packages of behavioural or psychological interventions and consolidate those aspects of nursing and family practitioner care which are already delivering such interventions in principle, as a formal part of primary care training and work. This is not a new idea, but it remains controversial with psychologists, who, like everyone in such situations, do not wish to see their professional skills undermined or diluted. It is being pioneered in primary care treatment of low back pain and Kleinman, for example,[16] points to this as an underexplored area of pain management. There is a real need for larger, better trials of this type of approach.

The same arguments apply to other aspects of the 'package' – return to work, education, exercise programmes. There is a need to develop practical packages, but to retain choice and therapists' individuality, at the same time as testing out the packages and establishing how often brief interventions may need to be reinforced to effectively reduce both the severity and the risk of persistence and recurrence.

These proposals bring two other implications for the future. First is the need for a very broad common set of skills among therapists treating chronic musculoskeletal pain. The end of the twentieth century saw official moves in the UK towards enabling a whole range of health professionals to prescribe drugs. This is part of an extension of the role of professionals such as pharmacists and nurses into areas such as chronic pain management, which is likely to continue and which will involve a range of skills far broader than drug prescription. The attraction of this is the development of a broader and better pain management profession. The danger is that the specific skills which make a physiotherapist a physiotherapist and not a nurse for example will be lost, and these may be the explicit skills which patients seek out, because they provide choice and give confidence. This leads to the second point. Patients are likely to have growing influence on the nature and content of chronic pain management programmes. If choice and expectation and goal setting have important beneficial effects on chronic pain, then harnessing patient involvement can be seen as a positive step, not only in its own right but also as a real contribution to more effective pain management.

What is left for the doctor to manage?

The role of the doctor in managing chronic musculoskeletal pain must change. The frustrations and iatrogenesis of the twentieth century must be replaced by overturning the old biomedical models, returning to the central notion of care,[17] and embracing new approaches to pain management supported by the ideas from pain neurobiology.

The story of surgery provides an example. Leriche, a French surgeon of the earlier twentieth century is, quite justifiably, applauded in Rey's history of pain[10] because he battled against the common view that pain was there to be suffered rather than relieved. He is also applauded however for making pain surgery the cornerstone of the ethical stance – the urgency to fight pain gives the clarion call for more surgery an ethical dimension. An extension to Rey's account reviewed postwar advances and pointed out that Leriche's ideas had become symbolic only, important because of his refusal to accept pain as a necessary evil, but lacking substance since the actual contribution of surgery was very limited. We leave the twentieth century with low back referrals to hospital being managed by physiotherapists and clinicians and the multidisciplinary team, and only a marginal look-in for the surgeons. The idea of surgery as a last gasp treatment for chronic pain (sever the nerve or disrupt connections in the cortex, for example) is now proven to be a problem. It disturbs the equilibrium and, as the neurobiology highlights, plasticity does not always take kindly to such crude attempts to halt the pain. It is likely that surgery will be increasingly discredited as a treatment for chronic musculoskeletal pain without a clear underlying pathology.

The surgical baby however must not be thrown away. The replacement of joints diseased with osteoarthritis is the outstanding success story of chronic musculoskeletal pain management from the past 50 years. The surgical treatment of injuries is likely to improve and continue to influence the prevention of chronic pain. And a clever series of experiments showing how local anaesthesia directed at peripheral sites of injury relieved the pain of chronic whiplash injury highlighted the fact that the next decades of unravelling the practical implications of the neurobiology of pain may lead us back to peripheral mechanisms of processing pain as much as to the central nervous system.[18]

Will organisation of care change?

The case for better management of acute pain as a means to prevent chronic musculoskeletal pain is strong. The insights from neurobiology point to the early development of chronic changes within an acute pain episode and suggest that the timeframe is short. Chronicity is not a late reaction to acute pain – the seedbed is there as an integral part of a pain episode from the start. Efficient immediate therapy may reduce the potential for chronicity – here new drugs and new methods of delivery of those drugs can help. The huge changes which the past two decades have seen in operative analgesia and the treatment of cancer pain have shown what can be done with organisation of care when a problem is taken seriously.

Current approaches to back pain present a similar revolution with the shift from primary care responses which encouraged the patient to immobilise their spine and which referred on to a surgeon, to more active approaches such as early activity and avoidance of bed rest. Yet a recent UK government report concluded that specialist services for acute pain in hospitals were still poorly organised, showed much variation and lacked dedicated nurse and doctor input.[19] More tellingly from the point of view of musculoskeletal pain is that good practice is currently focused on postoperative pain. Management of injury in trauma departments for example was not given the same priority. Although it requires research to demonstrate effectiveness, optimal treatment of acute pain and injury in the community and in hospitals is likely to lead to a reduction in chronic pain syndromes.

In the 1960s Cicely Saunders started the hospice movement, aware that care of the dying patient left much to be desired, and in particular pain relief for the cancer sufferer needed radical change. By 1978 a medical journalist could write of his pessimism that allocation of hospital services for pain management which "could be introduced almost overnight"[20] were unlikely because of "conservatism and a shortage of National Health Service funds". He quoted a study by the British Pain Society which concluded that "every district hospital should have a specialist on its staff offering two or three sessions per week for dealing with chronic pain cases, and regional or teaching hospitals should have preferably two clinicians with supporting staff devoted to the problems of pain".

By the year 2000, the Clinical Standards Advisory Group in the UK[19] was able to conclude that "palliative care services, providing pain relief for many patients with cancer, are generally focused and well organised, with specialist nurses educating other professionals. However, funding is often provided by charities and reductions in NHS spending were reported." They found that 86% of acute NHS trusts (the current equivalent of the district hospital) had a chronic pain service, but "the level and nature of provision varies markedly within the UK" and the services were "so poorly resourced that many could not meet local need... shortages of specialist chronic pain nurses, psychology, physiotherapy, occupational therapy and pharmaceutical support... hospital trust boards were reluctant to consider increased funding". This is in the context of a review of effectiveness of a chronic pain service which, whilst highlighting the need for more empirical evidence, concluded that they do offer a cost effective service.

What does this indicate for the future? It shows that some things have changed in the course of the past 25 years and that care for cancer patients in pain and provision of some chronic pain services reflect the possibility for improvement. However, it also highlights the continuing poor resourcing of pain services, the dramatic regional variations, and the large shortfall in providing effective pain management even with the tools and methods currently available. Closing this gap, reducing variation and improving resources, are achievable targets for the next decade – these are political, organisational and educational goals that require no new technologies or therapeutic advances. It might not be so exciting as the magic bullet, but it would be my best bet for an achievable goal that would improve the care of people in chronic musculoskeletal pain.

However, the major shift that must occur is to bring the focus of attention for the management of chronic musculoskeletal pain into primary care and away from hospitals. The new understanding of pain encourages broader skills in pain management across a range of professionals, a reduced obsession with the old pathology-led diagnosis as the route to effective therapy, and an emphasis on early and effective active pain management as a route to preventing chronicity. These all imply that primary care should be developed to lead, organise and deliver pain management.

Will the cultural perspective on chronic pain change?

Reading the chronic pain literature of the past decade, it is clear that one view at least is uniformly held, regardless of whether neural fibres or psyche hold the key to the secrets of the problem: a shared attitude that pain patients deserve similar investment of time, resource, effort and belief, regardless of cause. Respect for the patient in chronic pain has increased, with general agreement that malingering is rare and that the pain patient above all is searching for the pain to be taken seriously and believed.

Yet this is not necessarily the case in current routine primary care or rheumatology, and it is understandable why. Kleinman has written eloquently of the "duet of escalating antagonism" which arises as both sides of the clinical fence in a pain consultation get frustrated at the lack of a diagnosis that could help them both out of this hole.[16] The demands and obsessions of patients in chronic pain can seem unreasonable to hard-pressed doctors, with the disinterestedness or helplessness of the doctors equally unreasonable to the patient.

A major advance would surely be for changes in the culture of pain to lead to an acceptance on both sides that classic pathology is not the answer and that classic ideas of cure will not provide panaceas. Different goals and targets are needed, although good pain relief is an essential part of this.

The biggest frustration for rheumatologists and patients is the "pain without obvious cause", whether it is focussed on a specific area such as the back, or is more diffuse such as fibromyalgia. Such syndromes are tied up particularly with the general influences on chronicity such as anxiety, fear and depression. Some authors are tempted to bracket them as exclusively psychological cases and as only about psychology, a move equally reductionist as saying that there must be an underlying muscle or spine pathology to explain it. As pointed out earlier, such a move does not necessarily lead to better management. Simply because there is a psychological component to a pain does not mean that a purely psychological treatment is the most effective way to manage it. A sympathetic physiotherapist carrying out back massage or manipulation may be as effective for some people's distress as seeing a psychologist.

The compromise to this "mind–body" problem lies in the neurobiological story we now have which supports the continuing recognition of the reality of subjectively expressed pain. This should help to change medical culture that pain is only "real" when there is a test of abnormal local pathology available.[9,17] Absurdities of twentieth century medicine, such as two surgeons in court arguing about the reality of someone else's pain, could disappear.

A more pessimistic view is that imaging of pain sensation in the brain will simply provide a different focus for the argument as to what is real pain or not. So, a particularly desirable advance would be the development of a liberalising language from the science of pain – one which does not polarise to "is this in the mind or in the body?" – but sees neural plasticity and its intimate involvement with psyche and society as being an elegant explanation of the reality of chronic pain rather than a notion dismissive of it.

An important cultural aspect of chronic pain syndromes, in richer countries at least, is the influence of the sickness benefits and invalidity schemes, dominated as they often are by such syndromes. Waddell has argued persuasively that the rising epidemic of chronic back pain seen in the past three decades is actually about the exponential rise in the rates of disability payments and early retirements associated with the problem.[7] Two pessimistic views of the future follow from that: such rates will continue to rise or governments will pretend they have solved the problem by altering welfare systems so that fewer are eligible for benefits. The optimistic view is that expectations in society will change as pain management becomes the goal, with the Holy Grail no longer cure but adaptation and active participation in life and work to an extent which meets individual expectations. To achieve this rather grand ideal will demand a job market that is actively involved in rehabilitation and adaptation to the needs of the chronic pain sufferer.

What then are the crucial cultural developments for the next decades? The capacity to develop a language and understanding of pain that will allow us to recognise and talk of its reality without recourse to crude pathological imperialism or psychological reductionism, and aided and informed by the new biology. The willingness to harness the power of non-specific, placebo and healer orientated medicines. I am pessimistic about the influence of profit and drug companies and the courts on the management of pain, but it would be good to be proven wrong.

Can chronic musculoskeletal pain be prevented?

Mortality from disease remains the main issue of political and public health. Globally this is important, and for individuals likewise. Mental illness is the UK's other major health target, again for understandable reasons. But if we are talking about impact on daily living and about human suffering, the epidemiology of pain indicates that musculoskeletal syndromes and their accompanying disability top the list of importance at a societal level.

The demography of the next 30 years, with a predicted 30% increase in the population of older people, will increase the burden of disability and suffering. Fries' classic article on future mortality trends raised two alternative futures: either increasing life expectancy and decline in mortality will mean a rising tide of morbidity, or the same fundamental changes which have brought about the decline in mortality will also influence morbidity into an inevitable decline. This debate is probably not relevant to chronic musculoskeletal pain. For, even if new cohorts are now healthier, nothing in our current knowledge suggests that crucial reductions in the chronic pain syndromes will occur. Furthermore the cultural and social science and epidemiological evidence suggest that there is a real rise in pain complaints beyond the release of morbidity from the upturned stone of mortality. Pain is here to stay.

But are there public health measures which will lead to a decline in musculoskeletal pain? Injuries – whether from road traffic accidents, sport or work – show little clear evidence of decline. This means that internationally countries where chronic musculoskeletal problems have traditionally had a lower profile, will have an increasing public health problem because of the powerful mixture of road traffic accidents and demographic change. Injuries at work – especially those arising from heavy lifting for example – should decline and may do so in the next 20 years, and this implies a reduction in the causes of longer-term musculoskeletal problems. The difficulty is not knowing the ergonomic effects – psychosocial as well as physical – of the new industries. Call centres and computers may carry just as much musculoskeletal baggage as the one hundred weight cornsacks of old, and within a potentially less amenable psychosocial environment.

To this must be added rising levels of obesity and declining rates of exercise. Deyo noted that large scale societal shifts in the frequency of musculoskeletal pain are more likely to come from the same broad changes that are needed to reduce coronary heart disease, such as improved exercise levels, reduced smoking, and weight control, than from targeted programmes of prevention among those in high risk industries for example.[21] This does fit with Fries' argument that improved morbidity will follow decline in incidence of the diseases which cause early mortality.[22] But apart from smoking reduction in some countries and social groups, the message is not good, and at the moment the decline in heart disease is coming about without those changes in lifestyle that might benefit musculoskeletal health. Far greater investment in physical activity seems the crucial shift, even at the risk of higher rates of acute exercise related injury.

To these factors must be added the effects of abuse, violence, war and torture. These have been too little explored in terms of their influence on long term musculoskeletal pain. Whether public or private, pain and injury inflicted under circumstances of extreme distress are likely to prove powerful explanations of later symptoms.

Chronic musculoskeletal pain may become the single commonest international public health problem as preventable fatal disease declines in incidence, even if it does not become the most important. The next decades will certainly reveal the mechanisms by which it develops. Whether prevention of chronicity focuses on social factors such as accidents and physical inactivity or on magic bullets aimed at specific points of our nervous systems, only time will tell. Either way, the coming together of healers and neurobiologists, patients and doctors, traditional and complementary therapists, randomised controlled triallists and anthropologists, raises the hope that better understanding and treatments will emerge.

References

1 Wall P. *Pain: the science of suffering*. London: Phoenix Paperbacks, Orion Books Ltd, 2000.
2 Loeser JD, Melzack R. Pain: an overview. *Lancet* 1999;**353**:1607–9.
3 Besson JM. The neurobiology of pain. *Lancet* 1999;**353**:1610–15.
4 Roland M, van Tulder M. Should radiologists change the way they report plain radiography of the spine? *Lancet* 1998;**352**:229–30.
5 Raspe HH. Back pain. In: Silman AJ, Hochberg MC, eds. *Epidemiology of the rheumatic diseases*. Oxford: Oxford University Press, 1993;330–74.
6 Carr DB, Goudas LC. Acute pain. *Lancet* 1999;**353**:2051–58.
7 Waddell G. *The Back Pain Revolution*. Edinburgh: Churchill Livingstone, 1998.
8 Woolf CJ, Decosterd I. Implications of recent advances in the understanding of pain pathophysiology for the assessment of pain in patients. *Pain* 1999;(suppl 6):S141–7.
9 Morris DB. *The culture of pain*. Berkeley: University of California Press, 1991.
10 Rey R. *The history of pain*. Cambridge, MA: Harvard University Press, 1993.
11 Ashburn MA, Staats PS. Management of chronic pain. *Lancet* 1999;**353**:1865–69.
12 Willoughby DA, Moore AR, Colville-Nash PR. COX-1, COX-2, and COX-3 and the future treatment of chronic inflammatory disease. *Lancet* 2000;**355**:646–48.
13 Portenoy RK. Current pharmacotherapy of chronic pain. *J Pain Symptom Management* 2000;**19**:S16–20.
14 Turner JA, Deyo RA, Loeser JD, Von Korff M, Fordyce WE. The importance of placebo effects in pain treatment and research. *JAMA* 1994;**271**:1609–14.
15 Asher R. *Talking sense*. London: Pitman Medical, 1972.
16 Kleinman A. *Writing at the margin; the discourse between anthropology and medicine*. Berkeley: University of California Press, 1995.
17 Cassell EJ. Diagnosing suffering: a perspective. *Ann Int Med* 1999;**131**:531–4.
18 Lord SM, Barnsley L, Wallis BJ, Bogduk N. Chronic cervical zygapophysial joint pain after whiplash. *Spine* 1996;**21**:1737–45.
19 Clinical Standards Advisory Group. *Services for Patients with Pain*. London: Department of Health, 2000.

20 Fairley P. *The conquest of pain*. London: Michael Joseph, 1978.
21 Lahad A, Malter AD, Berg AO, Deyo RA. The effectiveness of four interventions for the prevention of low back pain. *JAMA* 1994;**272**:1286–91.
22 Fries JF. Aging, natural death and the compression of morbidity. *New Engl J Med* 1980;**303**:130–5.

8: The future diagnosis and management of trauma

BRUCE D BROWNER AND
ROSS A BENTHIEN

Introduction

Trauma to the musculoskeletal system encompasses a vast array of injuries, from sports related ligament sprains, to insufficiency fractures in the elderly and major long bone and pelvic fractures in high speed motor vehicle crashes. Trauma can also result in injury to joints, muscles, tendons, and other soft tissue that comprise the musculoskeletal system. Annually nearly 28 million Americans sustain 37 million traumatic injuries to the musculoskeletal system, representing a major portion of the total epidemiological distribution of musculoskeletal disorders (Table 8.1).[1] The cost of these traumatic

Table 8.1 Average annual episodes of injuries by type of injury, USA 1992–94 (adapted from Praemer et al.[1])

	Male	Female	Age (years)				Total
			L 18 y	18–44 y	45–64 y	65 y	
Fractures	3321	2625	1921	2344	777	904	5946
Dislocations/sprains	7121	6663	2746	7850	2174	1014	13784
Crush injuries	241	102	53	229	61	0	343
Open wounds	5060	2492	2152	3983	1009	408	7552
Contusions	2298	3103	1659	2635	751	986	6032
Other musculoskeletal injuries	1628	1616	919	1363	584	378	3244
Total musculoskeletal injuries	20299	16601	9450	18404	5356	3690	36901
Total injuries*	31159	26726	17117	26922	8034	5808	57885

*Numbers represent average annual episodes in thousands.
Includes injuries not listed in subcategories.

injuries represents a major portion of the 215 billion dollars (US$) spent on musculoskeletal conditions in the USA in 1995. This total included 89 billion in direct costs and 126 billion in indirect costs related to morbidity and mortality.[1]

Injuries are theoretically preventable but human nature, pervasive social and political factors, and even forces of nature make it inevitable that they will occur. The more profound injuries result in significant pain and disability and have high associated direct and indirect costs. While the efforts of orthopaedic surgeons have focussed on the treatment of injury, the greatest reductions in mortality and morbidity have been the byproduct of primary and secondary injury prevention programmes on the roads and in the workplace. These initiatives have produced a sustained reduction in injury in Western nations, but except in isolated cases have not been applied to the mushrooming industrial and transportation sectors of developing nations.

Any discussion of global injury prevention and treatment is often done on the basis of incomplete, inadequate or even non-existent information. Most countries in the world have developed some mechanism of compiling national information concerning deaths, but the collection of meaningful data about musculoskeletal injury is currently only possible in well developed market economies. Transferring lessons gleaned from this data to situations present halfway around the world in developing nations often does little to enlighten problems and potential solutions. With respect to injury, this effort is compromised by the absence of adequate national surveillance information from all countries. Standard data collection techniques used in developing countries may significantly underestimate the incidence of injury. Razzak and Luby showed that official sources of information on motor vehicle crashes captured only 56% of the fatalities and only 4% of the serious injuries in Karachi, Pakistan.[2] Standardised surveillance systems in all regions must be developed to allow better tracking of all types of injuries and permit the analysis of the effectiveness of prevention and treatment methods. Unanticipated events such as hurricanes, earthquakes, floods, wars and changing social trends could also have a major influence on the number of people injured in different parts of the world.

Even with complete information it is difficult to reliably predict future events beyond a horizon of a few years, and in the developing world prognostication takes the form of educated guesses. As a current exercise, we are looking at the next 10–20 years. Understanding the inherent limitations, an attempt has been made to discuss the evolving trends in musculoskeletal injury by subdividing them into causative mechanisms. In each case, factors influencing causation and prevalence are discussed. The challenges confronting developed and developing countries for prevention and treatment are then projected. Where appropriate, the impact of technological and scientific advances is considered.

Road traffic accidents

Overview

Annually, between 800 000 and 1 million people are killed, and approximately 23–34 million are injured or permanently disabled from accidents on the world's roads.[3] Between 75% and 85% of the fatalities and injuries occur in the developing world and the problem is growing. *The Global Burden of Disease and Injury*, a five-year study published in 1996 by researchers from the Harvard School of Public Health and the World Health Organization, examined the relative significance in terms of death and disability of the major health conditions and projected changes between 1990 and 2020.[4] A startling finding of this report was the prediction that road traffic accidents would move from ninth place to third place on the list as a cause of worldwide death and disability (measured in disability adjusted life years), exceeded only by ischaemic heart disease and unipolar major depression. By comparison, war is predicted to rank eighth and HIV tenth.[4] In its 1998 annual report, the International Federation of Red Cross and Red Crescent Societies (IFRC) recognised road traffic accidents as a major global health problem, compared in magnitude of seriousness to war and natural disasters.

Beginning in the 1970s, road safety improvements in North America, Europe, Japan, Australia, New Zealand and other developed countries resulted in significant reductions in the rates of motor vehicle fatalities and injuries mainly through the control of drunken driving and the mandatory use of child restraint devices and seatbelts. Additionally, improvements in passive protections, such as airbags and improved engineering of automotive passenger cabins, have further reduced the number of deaths and severity of injury. The result of these efforts are demonstrated in the United States Centers for Disease Control and Injury Prevention report, Healthy People 2010, that shows child seat use approaches 92% in children under age 4 and safety belt use in adults approaches 70%.[5] Unfortunately, these public safety initiatives have not been emphasised in developing countries. As motorised transport increases in developing nations, injury to unrestrained passengers will likely precipitate a public health crisis.

Causes

The global disparity in traffic safety related injuries are complex, but several causes have been identified. In highly motorised countries, the occupants of cars are the primary victims of traffic accidents. These nations have highly developed, mechanised transportation systems consisting of motor vehicles, trains and air travel, and proportionately less transportation is achieved through walking or two-wheeled transport. In the USA and Western Europe travellers are accustomed to travel on highways that are the product of intensive engineering, consistent repair and redundant passive safety structures. In addition, different modes of transportation are physically and temporally separated by barriers, traffic signals and elaborate traffic laws. In the developing world much the opposite is seen. Transportation in bustling cities is a dense mix of motorcycles, bicycles, pedestrians and livestock. Add to this sparse traffic safety laws and inadequate police enforcement and the ramifications become clear. Governments, not unexpectedly, focus on the efficient transport of goods from agricultural and manufacturing areas and modern safety features are often omitted.

The heterogeneous traffic stream seen in the developing world results in the troubling problem of vehicle mismatch. In the developing, newly motorised countries, vulnerable road users such as pedestrians, bicyclists, motorcycle and scooter riders, and passengers on public transportation sustain the majority of deaths and injuries. They travel together on the same roads with buses, trucks and cars in a chaotic traffic stream. Mismatched collisions between unprotected humans and the heavy vehicles cause frequent deaths and serious injury even at lower speeds.

This is clearly evidenced in Malaysia where 57% of traffic fatalities are related to motorised two wheeled transport and when pedestrian and bicycle fatalities are added the total jumps to 78%. By contrast, motorised four wheeled vehicles account for 79% of fatalities in the USA (Table 8.2).[6] A compendium of US travel safety data from 1990 demonstrated 37 081 fatalities were attributed to motor vehicle crashes; this compared to 856 related to bicycles and 6468 to

Table 8.2   Road users killed in various modes of transport (adapted from Global Traffic Safety Trust[6])

Location and year	Pedestrians	Bicyclists	Motorised two-wheelers	Motorised four-wheelers	Others
Delhi, India (1994)	42	14	27	12	5
Thailand (1987)	47	6	36	12	—
Bandung, Indonesia (1990)	33	7	42	15	3
Colombo, Sri Lanka (1991)	38	8	34	14	6
Malaysia (1994)	15	6	57	19	3
Japan (1992)	27	10	20	42	1
The Netherlands (1990)	10	22	12	55	—
Norway (1990)	16	5	12	64	3
Australia (1990)	18	4	11	65	2
USA (1995)	13	2	5	79	1

Numbers represent percentage of all road-related fatalities.

pedestrians. Motor vehicle accidents resulted in a fatality in less than 1% of accidents, compared to 3% for bicycles and 10% in pedestrians.[6] In the developed world it is clear the major culprit in road traffic related trauma is motor vehicles. A deeper look at the numbers cautions translating these observations to the very different situations seen in the developing world. In developing countries transportation growth is centred on two wheeled transport and pedestrian travel, not automobiles. Based on the high rate of fatalities from bicycle and pedestrian related accidents in the USA, road traffic accidents in the developing world (which involve more two-wheeled vehicles and pedestrians) most certainly results in significantly more deaths and morbidity. Data from the United States Centers for Disease Control published in the national public health blueprint, Healthy People 2010, shows that motor vehicle crashes result in 15.0 deaths and 1000 non-fatal injuries per 100 000 people. Pedestrian related accidents result in just 2.0 fatal and 29.0 non-fatal injuries per 100 000 people, again reflecting the emphasis on automobile transportation in the USA. A 30–50% reduction in these rates is the goal for the next decade.[5]

Unlike the developed countries where the cars are the predominant mode of private transportation, in the newly motorising countries, more affordable motorcycles and scooters are being purchased and

123

joining the unregulated traffic stream in large numbers. The resulting explosive 25–30% two wheeled power vehicle growth rate in many of the Asian countries will lead to doubling of the fleet in 5 years and tripling in 8 years, causing even more severe problems. This trend is clearly evident in Vietnam where 91% of vehicles are motorised two wheelers and only 9% are cars (Table 8.3).[6]

Table 8.3 Vehicle ownership by country (data from multiple sources, 1992–95; adapted from Global Traffic Safety Trust[6])

Country	GNP per capita	Total number of vehicles/1000 persons	MTWs* as percentage of total vehicles	Cars as a percentage of total vehicles
Japan	34630	640	20	58
USA	24780	740	2	88
Germany	23980	570	9	89
France	23420	520	10	87
UK	18340	410	3	86
Australia	18000	610	3	76
Republic of Korea	8260	206	24	33
Malaysia	3140	340	56	34
Thailand	2140	190	66	16
Philippines	950	32	26	28
Indonesia	810	58	69	15
Sri Lanka	600	50	60	13
China	530	21	40	24
India	320	30	67	14
Vietnam	210	27	91	9

*Motorised two-wheeler.

Societal impact

Traffic related trauma in the developed world, while diminishing, when added to the expected explosion in the newly developing world provides a significant challenge to the worldwide orthopaedic community. The Western experience with traffic related trauma predicts significant burdens on the health systems of developing countries, in many cases struggling to meet current health demands. The chronic absence of pre-hospital emergency care and limited resources for acute hospitalisation and rehabilitative care are additive factors explaining the increased morbidity and mortality from these accidents.

Along with the physical injuries related to this epidemic come significant economic and social consequences. The national economic impact of road crashes represents 0.5–4.0 of GNP depending on the country.[3] The World Bank estimates that the annual cost of traffic accidents is 500 billion dollars (US$) worldwide, with 100 billion dollars (US$) in cost being attributed to the developing countries. As the combination of all forms of foreign loans and aid totals 60 billion dollars (US$), it is clear that road traffic accidents are seriously undermining the economic and social development in these countries.

Trauma victims are often young males who are the workers and wage earners in their families. When they are killed or disabled, there is a profound effect on their entire family. In some countries, unfavourable customs and laws do not provide for support of the widows and families of those killed and the accident leads also to the break up of the family. The enormous volume of suffering and disability, and the magnitude and impact of economic costs of road traffic injuries in the economic world, qualify them as an epidemic and demands a definitive response from the world community.

Prevention

Decades of experience in Western countries has shown that successful prevention of road traffic injuries cannot be accomplished with single measures, requiring instead simultaneous initiatives in the areas of education, enforcement, engineering, environment and emergency medicine. There is much technical expertise and experience with these modalities that could be shared with the newly motorising countries. The governments, non-governmental organisations, and professional and technical communities must recognise road traffic injuries as a major public health problem and foreign policy issue, and give the highest priority to activities in this area. The United Nations, World Health Organization and International Federation of Red Cross and Red Crescent Societies must lend their support to appropriately structured focused programmes. Loans would be available from the World Bank, but developing countries' governments must become officially interested in this problem to request loans for road traffic injury prevention and treatment programmes. A new spirit of volunteerism amongst healthcare professionals and technical personnel in Organization for Economic Cooperation and Development countries must be stimulated so that they will spend time working with their counterparts in developing countries to develop sustainable expertise.

The rate of road traffic accidents has begun to plateau and fall in most developed countries. Continued technological advancements in automotive design will further improve occupant protection and crash avoidance. Incorporation of computer technology into roads will improve traffic separation and further reduce accidents. Competition among automakers in developed market economies will spread these technical advances from the high end vehicles through the rest of the fleet to the less expensive models. To reduce the costs of vehicles, those manufactured in developing countries do not contain standard safety features provided by major new manufacturers. Over the next two decades, the opening of major new markets such as China may allow for the introduction of large numbers of cars where very few had previously been purchased. This will offer an opportunity but an economic challenge to ensure that the new fleets developed will contain essential safety features.

Prehospital care

Modern trauma care in the USA and Western Europe relies on a highly technological and resource intensive system of prehospital care based on a vast communication and transportation infrastructure. Ambulances transport patients on an extensive high speed highway system, and in many communities helicopters provide rapid transport to care facilities. In addition, generous government support in the decades following the second world war produced thousands of highly trained medical professionals and hospitals. Patients injured in motor vehicle crashes, especially in urban centres, receive thorough trauma care often within minutes of the accident. The continuous evolution of emergency medical services in developed countries has been an important mechanism to decrease death and disability following road traffic accidents. Standardised training of emergency medical technicians and paramedics, medical supervision and communications, and ambulance and helicopter transport have all been important aspects of systems development. Public access has generally been facilitated through special telephone numbers such as 911. The timely response of ambulance and field personnel has been legislated by local authorities. These systems are often not present in developing countries. Injured patients are often transported by informal arrangements with truckers and bus drivers. To improve this situation, police and commercial transporters should be trained as medical first-responders. Subsequent emergency medical systems can be developed following the urban and rural models utilised in developed countries. While models for efficient trauma care exist, the lacking transportation and medical infrastructure in the developing world make technology transfer a difficult proposition.

Treatment

Trauma centres have played an important role in improving the care of serious injuries resulting from road traffic accidents and other causes in the developed countries. Adoption of the facilities and medical staff models of these units is usually possible only in major cities in developing countries. In the more peripheral areas, district hospitals are staffed only by general medical officers or general surgeons. Specialised orthopaedic trauma training must be developed for these individuals to be better prepared to care for frequent victims of road traffic accidents. Programmes such as Orthopaedics Overseas, World Orthopaedic Concern, International Red Cross and Red Crescent, and a variety of Christian missionary groups have developed successful models for sending volunteers to work at district hospitals. This type of programme should be expanded. In addition to recruiting additional volunteers and expanding programme sites, specialised educational materials for road traffic injury care in the developing world must be developed.

Surgical techniques for treating fractures in virtually every anatomical location have been developed. External fixation, plating and intramedullary nailing techniques have been refined over the last 20 years. Recently, the emphasis has been placed on introducing implants with minimally invasive techniques; utilising specially designed implants and instrumentation, radiographic guidance with fluoroscopy, indirect fracture reduction and implant insertion through much smaller incisions. By eliminating surgical dissection, secondary trauma has been reduced, resulting in less infection and more predictable and rapid healing. In the future, more sophisticated intraoperative radiographic guidance with such techniques as computed tomography will allow even greater levels of precision, insertion of implants in more challenging anatomical locations with even less surgical invasion.

High energy injury which produces bone loss and healing problems may be overcome with the introduction of genetically engineered bone morphogenic proteins, bioabsorbable carrier materials and bone graft substitutes. Some of these products are already on the market and others are nearing the final phases of clinical testing and will soon be released. Electrical stimulation which has been utilised for two decades and low intensity ultrasound, which was released more recently, must be studied scientifically to determine if they are effective adjuncts to accelerate fracture union. Continued investigation over the next 20 years may result in the discovery, testing and market introduction of new materials that will supplant currently used metallic fracture fixation implants.

Lack of surgical sophistication and the lack of basic operating room asepsis and technical capability make the option of internal fixation methods impossible at the district hospital level in developing countries. The first step would be the introduction of external fixation. This would make it possible to salvage some open fractures of the upper and lower extremity which are currently treated by amputation. Successful adoption of this technique and improvement of the operating room environment would provide a basis for introducing methods of internal fixation. At present, the cost of implants utilised in the developed market economies is well beyond the economic capabilities in the developing countries. Simplified, affordable effective implants and effective instrumentation will have to be developed before these techniques can be employed. Until this is possible, functional bracing and orthotic technology should be imported. Many fractures can be treated with inexpensive prefabricated plastic braces. This would represent an improvement over current therapy resulting in reduction of deformity and disability.

While urban centres enjoy leading edge trauma care, rural America still faces a significant disparity in quality trauma care. Only one third of the US population resides in a rural location but they incur nearly 57% of the motor vehicle trauma related deaths. This disparity is due to delay in discovering victims, longer transport times to, or lack of, trauma facilities and the skill of prehospital care providers.[7] Improving survival for rural citizens of motor vehicle trauma will require increased resources for training of prehospital care personnel, improved triage systems and air transport to level one trauma centres.

War injuries

Overview

War related injuries to combat personnel and the civilian population continue to be significant sources of musculoskeletal trauma worldwide. While peace agreements are being signed in many areas of the world that have been plagued with constant conflict, such as Northern Ireland and the Balkans, conflict continues throughout the world and new regional conflicts are sure to develop over the next 20 years. The power and accuracy of military weapons continues to increase and a modern consequence of war is the increasing mortality and morbidity sustained by civilians during wartime. In the first world war, civilians accounted for no more than 19% of all war related deaths, that number jumped to 48% in the second world war, and to 80% in recent conflicts.[8] The introduction of biological chemical or tactical nuclear weapons can further complicate the care of injuries including those in the musculoskeletal system.

Land mines

When addressing war related musculoskeletal trauma, land mines deserve special mention. Estimates from the International Committee of the Red Cross and the United States State Department are that 90–120 million antipersonnel land mines are deployed throughout the world and 2.5 million new mines are planted each year.[9,10] Soldiers that are not killed but sustain major injury to their lower extremities often require amputation. Continued improvements in military boots and uniforms may mitigate some of these injuries but the ingenuity of land mine designers will surely blunt the value of any protective advantage.

The worldwide carnage from land mines continues to inflict devastating losses on inhabitants of rural communities long after armed conflict has ended. These devices remain active in the ground for long periods, often decades, providing prolonged, potentially catastrophic exposure to local inhabitants. Attempts by indigenous people to reclaim the land for agriculture leads to frequent detonations resulting in many civilian deaths and serious musculoskeletal injuries. Sadly, children are frequently the victims of these devices. A study of 206 communities in Afghanistan, Bosnia, Cambodia and Mozambique showed that between 25% and 87% of households had daily activities affected by land mines. Overall 6% of households reported a land mine victim, one third of the encounters were fatal and 1 in 10 involved children. These injuries and death have serious economic implications including care of the injured and loss of labour for farming. Households with a land mine victim were 40% more likely to have difficulty providing food.[11] During a one month period in the summer of 1999, 150 people were injured or killed in Kosovo from landmines for an annual rate of 120 per 100 000. Most of the victims were men and boys, with 71% younger than 24 years of age.[12]

Countries such as Angola, Afghanistan, Cambodia, Mozambique, Kosovo, Sudan, Laos, Iraq and Vietnam have the highest density of devices and the most injuries. This problem has only recently been identified and actively addressed as an international public health concern. The public health community must still work to define the scope and magnitude of the problem, identify those at risk for injury by occupation or demographics, and finally evaluate and implement interventions.[13]

Since these devices are inexpensive, and active war zones still exist, far more are placed in the ground each week than are removed. These devices are designed to be undetectable by trained enemies and local authorities encounter significant difficulty clearing them after conflict is over. Currently, a painstaking and expensive process is required to remove each land mine. They must be located with a probe stick and carefully evacuated by hand. Twenty-two percent of victims were injured during attempted removal of these devices.

Those who survive inevitably end up with amputations. In Cambodia one of every 236 people is an amputee and in Afghanistan nearly 1 in 50 people is a victim of land mines.[14] The demand for acute orthopaedic care and the prolonged rehabilitation and prosthetic needs of this population surely far exceeds the capabilities of the local health system. A child undergoing traumatic amputation of a limb would require dozens of prostheses over an average life expectancy. The difficulty in addressing this need is emphasised by the fact that only 1 in 8 amputees in Cambodia have a prosthetic limb.[9]

Prevention

As for any other public health crisis, primary prevention is the most efficacious and least expensive form of intervention. Modern military strategy and equipment provides soldiers with effective protection from injury and death. As a result civilian injury and death represents the vast majority of war related trauma. Therefore intervention strategies should address the vulnerability of civilian populations. Clearly the most efficacious intervention would be the peaceful resolution of world conflicts and the avoidance of war. Further interventions would work to prevent the worldwide sale and proliferation of arms and making what arms that are sold less lethal (and understandably less desirable). Spatially removing civilians from combat zones through the establishment of safe havens or pre-emptive evacuations would mitigate civilian losses. Other effective but more expensive interventions would provide civilians with barrier protections including helmets, flack jackets, gas masks, reinforced living quarters, and sheltered public market and water sources.[8]

Prevention of land mine related injuries has received increased attention recently. The situation will only be reversed by an international ban on the devices or the introduction of time limited fuses. Over 120 nations have signed the Convention on the Prohibition of the Use, Stockpiling, Production and Transfer of Anti-Personnel Landmines and on their Destruction, while far fewer have ratified the provisions of the document. In the future, new technologies may develop which will allow devices currently in place to be detected. Alternatively, sonic waves or robots could be used to explode the devices and reclaim areas of land for agricultural use.

Prehospital care

Caring for combat personnel with musculoskeletal injuries presents increased challenges compared to similar civilian injuries. Hot or tropical climates such as the desert or the jungle can further complicate open musculoskeletal injuries, leading to a higher incidence of wound infection and osteomyelitis. Mountainous terrain and limited capability for air transport, such as that experienced by the Russian army in Afghanistan, could interfere with early first aid for open fractures and the timely transport of injured soldiers. Well funded military development projects may lead to advances in wound care and acute injury management. The military is particularly interested in the use of telemedicine, teleradiology and distant robotic surgery. Extensive funding for such government programmes allows opportunities for technological development, which can then be transferred to the civilian sector. Military surgeons can also improve the care of soldiers with musculoskeletal injuries by adopting advances in intraoperative image guidance, implant and instrument design, and fracture healing enhancements.

Treatment

The vast majority of injuries from land mines are to the lower extremities. Data from 587 civilian, war related injuries in Sri Lanka demonstrated that a majority, 349, resulted from land mines: the lower extremities were involved in nearly half the cases; 23% underwent amputation, and 84% of these were below the knee.[15] While modern orthopaedic trauma principles advocate surgical irrigation and debridement of these wounds within six hours of injury, this is inherently difficult in the developing world. Estimates are that only 28% of land mine victims receive hospital care within six hours of injury, increasing the risk of shock and limb threatening infection. The International Committee of the Red Cross has described three injury categories related to antipersonnel mines. Pattern 1 involves traumatic amputation of the lower extremity from stepping on a device. Pattern 2 usually results from detonation of the device near a victim with fewer injuries to the extremities, but torso injuries are more prevalent. Finally, pattern 3 injuries occur from handling mines during disarmament and results in severe upper extremity and facial injuries.[16] The effects on limb salvage rates and functional outcomes of these higher energy injuries within the disordered healthcare delivery systems seen in war-torn regions or developing nations is certain to lead to excess morbidity. Efforts at identifying these injuries early and providing standard treatment algorithms in specialised centres should increase the rate of limb salvage.

Fragility fractures

The epidemiology and causative factors of fragility fractures are discussed in Chapter 6 on osteoporosis and will not be repeated here. It is worth re-emphasising, however, the number of hip fractures worldwide requiring hospitalisation, and surgical treatment is growing at a rate that is greater than the ageing of the population. In the USA, adults aged 65 or older account for 88% of all healthcare expenditures for fractures resulting from loss of bone density. Excess healthcare costs for the year following hip fracture are estimated at $15 000 (US$) with aggregate of $2.9 billion in the entire Medicare population aged 65 or over.[17] In the next 15–20 years, the baby boomers will reach retirement. If research and public health measures do not dramatically alter the prevalence of osteoporosis, there will be an enormous increase in hip fractures and other fragility fractures. Estimates are that by 2040, 512 000 hip fractures per year could occur with estimated costs of $16 billion (in 1984 dollars).[17] This represents a roughly 70% increase from 300 000 hip fractures currently treated in the USA. Finnish researchers have demonstrated an increase in the incidence of hip fractures from 163 (per 100 000 population) in 1970 to 438 in 1997. Even when age adjusted, the rate in men increased from 112 to 233 and in women from 292 to 467. If these trends continue, a tripling of the number of hip fractures will be seen by 2030.[18] While hip fractures are the most resource intensive fragility fracture, compression fractures of the spine, wrist fractures and humerus fractures all affect the osteopenic elderly in disproportionate numbers. While femur fractures often result from high energy injuries sustained by the young, as many as 25% occur in elderly women from low energy falls.[19]

Senior citizens in many countries of the world are adopting increasingly active lifestyles, including travel and sporting activities. These individuals are sustaining injuries to various locations in the skeleton. The osteoporosis makes their bones thinner and more brittle. Fractures are associated with greater degrees of fragmentation. These two factors make fracture fixation much more challenging. Orthopaedic surgeons and traumatologists are already searching for new methods of achieving fixation in osteoporotic bone. Current techniques involve augmentation with bone cement. In the future, new implants and materials will be developed to facilitate this therapy.

There is increasing recognition that the outcome of treating hip fractures is dependent on careful recognition and management of the many associated medical problems which present in these elderly individuals. The one year mortality rate after hip fracture is increased compared to matched controls, and recent reports by the American Academy of Orthopaedic Surgeons highlights the continued problems in this area. The team approach, which incorporates orthopaedic surgeons, internal medicine physicians, cardiologists, geriatricians, nurses, physical therapists, nutritionists and social workers, has given improved results. In coming years, this approach will have to be further refined and spread to all countries. Studies of the principal medical specialties show that primary care doctors, internists and orthopaedic surgeons are not routinely performing adequate screening, prevention and treatment of osteoporotic patients. Programmes will have to be initiated to change professional behaviour. To make these possible, governments will have to recognise the value of these initiatives and provide adequate reimbursement of medical services for the prevention and treatment of osteoporosis. In addition to primary intervention, patients who have sustained fragility fractures will have to be referred to primary care physicians and specialists for the treatment of osteoporosis and multifactorial fall prevention to avoid subsequent fractures.

Industrial and agricultural injuries

Machinery utilised in manufacturing, construction and agriculture has great potential to produce injuries to the musculoskeletal system. In developed market economies, these injuries have been markedly reduced by occupational safety laws, which are administrated by national agencies. After many years of implementation, these laws have led to important safety features being incorporated into machines and the work setting. Restrictions on child labour have also helped to reduce this type of injury. These laws and their oversight agencies do not exist in most developing countries. Globalisation of markets and the development of many international corporations have been associated with shifting of manufacturing to developing countries, where low labour costs, favourable tax structure, and limited environmental and safety regulations reduce overheads and enhance profit margin. Growing manufacturing centres have caused the migration of farm workers from the countryside to growing mega-cities in search of better employment. Long hours, dangerous working conditions and abusive labour practices produce the ideal setting for frequent work related injuries. Although these countries benefit from the economic growth associated with importation of manufacturing, governments must be encouraged to adopt environmental protection and workers' safety regulations. Standards found in developed market economies must be implemented in developing countries to protect the environment and ensure human rights. These regulations will avoid many serious injuries, which would otherwise require expensive medical care. Together with road traffic injuries, work related injuries consume health resources.

A recent emphasis has been placed on the health and safety of child labourers. While much media attention has focussed on deplorable working conditions for children in regions of the developing world, the United States Centers for Disease Control has showed that the workplace can be hazardous for children in the USA. Estimates are that 2.6 million 16 and 17 year old adolescents work at least part time. These numbers do not reflect younger workers often employed in agriculture.[20] In 1993, the Bureau of Labor Statistics in a survey of 250 000 private business establishments identified over 20 000 injuries and illnesses in children, 18% were contusions, 16% were sprains and 4% were fractures or dislocations.[20] About 300 youths die each year from farm-related injuries, and 23500 suffer non-fatal injuries. Data from a survey of Iowa farms showed that 40% of children operated machinery unsupervised and the average age at which they started operation was 12. Nearly 50% of the victims of fatal injuries die prior to reaching a physician, re-emphasising the continued shortcomings present in rural trauma care.[21]

While tractors cause the majority of fatal farm accidents, only 5–10% of non-fatal injuries are related to tractors. Only one third of tractors on US farms are equipped with seat belts and antirollover devices and the rates are much lower in the developing world.[21] As mechanisation of crop production and processing increases throughout the world the frequency and severity of orthopaedic trauma related to this industry will increase.

Sports injuries

In developed market economies, participation in competition and recreational athletics results in a large number of ligament sprains, muscle strains and fractures. While most of these problems would be classified as minor, they often require medical care and do result in some limited loss of work time and interference with other activities. By sheer numbers, they become significant in their social and economic impact. A number of current trends will expand over the next two decades to make these problems even more significant.

The combination of genetic evolution and physical conditioning is producing athletes that are larger, stronger and faster. Despite improvements in protective equipment, these factors will produce larger numbers of severe injuries, particularly in contact sports. While the types of sports related injuries are numerous and nearly every portion of the musculoskeletal system can be affected, focussing on anterior cruciate ligament injuries may highlight some key issues and demographics. The incidence of acute anterior cruciate ligament injuries in the USA is estimated at between 80000 and 100000 per year and the cost of related treatment is estimated at 1 billion dollars (US$). The highest incidence of injury occurs in young men aged 15–25 involved in pivoting sports. The majority of anterior cruciate ligament injuries occur in men and result from non-contact mechanisms. Current research is actively investigating the rate of these anterior cruciate ligament injuries specifically, and musculoskeletal injuries in general in female athletes in comparison to their male counterparts. Data published by the National Collegiate

Athletic Association (NCAA) from their injury surveillance programme showed a higher rate of anterior cruciate ligament injury compared to men in both soccer and basketball.[22] Similar investigations at the United States Naval Academy showed that female midshipmen had a 2.44 relative risk of sustaining an anterior cruciate ligament injury. Women had a higher relative risk of being injured in intercollegiate sports (3.96), military training (9.74) and in coed sports (1.40).[23] Multiple factors have been described to explain the observed differences including anatomical, increased joint laxity, hormonal, muscle strength and knee stiffness, and jumping and landing characteristics.[24] No clear aetiology has yet been demonstrated, but active research continues.

The current generation of thrill seeking youths has created and popularised new "extreme sports". Group skydiving, sky surfing, roller blading, snow boarding, street luge, bungee jumping, mountain biking and free climbing are a few examples of these new activities. Undoubtedly, the next two decades will witness the development of even more challenging and injury threatening sports. Austrian researchers looked at the incidence of snowboarding related injuries and collected data on over 2500 snowboarders. They found 152 injuries, with 107 requiring medical treatment. The corresponding injury was 10.6 per 1000 snowboarding days, with the rate of moderate to severe injuries 5.4 per 1000 days. The upper extremity was injured in 61% of cases, with the wrist the most frequently injured site. Lack of experience increases the risk of injury, while the use of wrist protection devices resulted in a significant reduction in injuries.[25] This is compared to a longer history of skiing related injury data showing 2.5 injuries per 1000 skier-days. Many feel this number underestimates the true incidence of 4–5 per 1000 skier-days. Women and children appear to be at higher risk for skiing related injuries.[26] While similar numbers can be developed for the wide variety of sports activities people participate in, as women continue to swell the ranks of sport participators and as modernisation of the developing world provides more opportunity to participate in sports the incidence of these injuries will increase. In addition, as personal wealth increases, people will increasingly seek treatment for sports related injuries, or other musculoskeletal conditions that interfere with performance.

Continuing incorporation of computer technology and robotics into manufacturing, shipping and agriculture will simplify work and produce more leisure time. Economic growth in additional areas of the world will expand the middle class and increase involvement in these sporting activities. Shorter workweeks, earlier retirement and the adoption of increasingly active lifestyles will dramatically expand the number of people who will sustain musculoskeletal injuries while participating in sports and recreational activities. The current emphasis on physical fitness will expand. Although the physical condition and the health status of the population will improve, excessive functional expectations of older individuals will cause many to exceed the physical tolerance of their soft tissues. Treatment and rehabilitation of sports injuries in senior citizens will become a special challenge.

There is a growing expectation among persons of all ages that they will recover from their sports injuries and return to both competitive and recreational sports within a very short period of time. Because of the intense interest in this area, there is enormous potential for fraud and economic abuse. Increased funding and research will have to be devoted to accurately determine the best methods to accomplish these goals.

Competitive overuse and cumulative stress injuries

This is a special category for industrial injuries. Motions, which involve power pinch and wrist flexion, such as those utilised by arbetoirs in the poultry industry or clerical workers who perform keyboarding, produce a classic carpal tunnel syndrome. This problem has been well recognised in advanced market economies and is generally avoided by work redesign, ergonomics and early treatment. These lessons will have to be observed in the developing countries to which many industries in which workers utilise repetitive motions have been transferred. These work related illnesses appear to be on the decline in the USA, but as the developing world turns to more mechanised agriculture and manufacturing, the potential for an increasing global burden of work related illnesses is clear.

The Bureau of Labor Statistics surveys US businesses yearly to assess the type and severity of workplace related illnesses. A 1994 sampling of 250 000 private sector businesses yielded over 700 000 cases of overexertion or repetitive motion. Overexertion resulted in 530 000 injuries, the majority affecting the back. Just over 90 000 injuries were related to repetitive motion, the majority of these affecting the wrist. Over 30 studies have evaluated the relationship between carpal tunnel syndrome and work. There is convincing evidence that carpal tunnel syndrome is related to highly repetitive, forceful and vibratory work activities. The relationship is stronger when these factors are combined in work activities. A review of eight studies evaluating hand and wrist tendinitis arrived at similar conclusions. Hand–arm vibration syndrome is a constellation of vascular related symptoms from the use of jackhammers, chainsaws and similar equipment. Strong evidence supports that the intensity and duration of exposure is related to the development of these disorders. A review of over 40 studies of low back disorders and physical workplace factors supports evidence for heavy physical work and awkward postures as causative agents. Strong evidence of association was demonstrated for work related lifting, forceful movements and whole body vibration. The lifetime prevalence of low back pain is 70% in industrialised nations and accounts for 16% of worker's compensation claims and 33% of costs. Growing evidence demonstrates that a number of psychosocial factors are related to the incidence of these syndromes, including job dissatisfaction, intensified workloads, monotonous work, job control, job clarity and social support.[27]

Orthopaedic surgeons and primary care providers are asked to evaluate and treat these patients on a routine basis, often for extended periods of time. While operative interventions are undertaken for the minority of patients, the direct and indirect costs in lost productivity, disability and medical intervention are enormous. As industrialisation of the world progresses, the incidence of these disorders is sure to increase and will further tax healthcare systems already overburdened by endemic disease and trauma. The statement of philosopher George Santiana, "Those who do not study history are doomed to repeat it", applies well to this situation. Failure to implement the prevention and treatment methods established by the developed market economies after years of experience will condemn the developing countries to repetition of large numbers of these complaints. In these cases, chronic pain results from microscopic injury to muscles and tendons due to accumulative overstress. The problem can also be managed by work redesign, ergonomic improvements and conditioning. As computers proliferate to all areas of the world for personal and business use, the problem will become more widespread. In coming years, it is expected that evolutions in the design of computers and workstations will decrease this problem. As economic factors always delay the incorporation of new technology, this problem may be seen in developing countries before they are able to afford newer equipment. The proper diagnosis and treatment of this syndrome is still controversial even in the developed market economies.

Summary

Taken together all the mechanisms discussed above and natural phenomenon such as earthquakes and hurricanes will produce millions of musculoskeletal injuries over the next 10–20 years. Special attention needs to be given to the problem of road traffic accidents. Left uncontrolled, injuries from this cause alone will consume 25% of the health budget in many developing countries by the year 2010. At the present rate, road traffic injuries will grow to become the third leading cause of death and disability by the year 2020. Current scientific advances and future technical developments will further enhance our ability to diagnose and treat bone and soft tissue injuries. New advances will enhance and accelerate the healing of these tissues. Governments, non-government organisations, healthcare providers and technical personnel from developed market economies will have to help their counterparts in developing countries to establish systems to prevent and treat many forms of musculoskeletal injury. The current efforts to achieve world peace and inactivate the weapons of war must be expanded. Ageing of the world's population will present new challenges in the treatment of fragility fractures. Lessons learned in the developed market economies with acute and cumulative work related injuries must be shared with developing countries to which many jobs are being shifted. Computers, economic prosperity and ageing of the world's population will expand the participation in sports and recreational activities. The creation of more demanding and dangerous sports will further expand the number of injuries. Each of these different types of injuries can be prevented by appropriate measures. Prevention is the most cost effective means of reducing the burden of injury. The disability and economic loss is associated with injuries that could be limited by the development of improved injury treatment by the establishment of adequate prehospital and hospital care in all countries of the world.

References

1 Praemer A, Furner S, Rice DP. *Musculoskeletal conditions in the United States.* American Academy of Orthopaedic Surgeons, 1999.
2 Razzak JA, Luby SP. Estimating deaths and injuries due to road traffic accidents in Karachi, Pakistan, through the capture–recapture method. *Int J Epidemiol* 1998;**27**:866–70.
3 Jacobs GD, Aeron-Thomas A, Astrop A. Estimating global road fatalities. Transport Research Laboratory, unpublished report, 1999.

4 Murray CJL, Lopez AD, eds. *The global burden of disease and injury.* Harvard School of Public Health and the World Health Organization, 1996.

5 Centers for Disease Control and Prevention and the National Institutes of Health. *Healthy People 2010*-Conference Edition, 1999.

6 Global Traffic Safety Trust. *Reflections on the transfer of traffic safety knowledge to motorising nations.* Melbourne, 1998.

7 Rodgers FB, Shackford SR, Osler TM, Vane DW, Davis JH. Rural trauma: the challenge for the next decade. *J Trauma* 1999;47:802–21.

8 Aboutanos MB, Baker SP. Wartime civilian injuries: epidemiology and intervention strategies. *J Trauma* 1997;43:719–26.

9 Hutson HR, Anglin D, Strote J. Antipersonnel land mines: why they should be banned. *Acad Emerg Med* 1998;5:205–8.

10 Anonymous. Landmine-related injuries, 1993–1996. *Morbidity & Mortality Weekly Report* 1997;46:724–6.

11 Andersson N, da Sousa CP, Paredes S. The social cost of land mines in four countries: Afghanistan, Bosnia, Cambodia, and Mozambique. *BMJ* 1995;311:718–21.

12 Krug EG, Gjini AA. Number of land mine victims in Kosovo is high. *BMJ* 1999;319(7207):450.

13 Krug EG, Ikeda RM, Qualls ML, Anderson MA, Rosenberg ML, Jackson, RJ. Preventing land mine-related injury and disability: a public health perspective. *JAMA* 1998;280:465–6.

14 Cobey J, Ayotte B. Tools to measure landmine incidents and injuries. *Lancet* 2000;355(9214):1549–50.

15 Meade P, Mirocha J. Civilian landmine injuries in Sri Lanka. *J Trauma* 2000;48:735–9.

16 Coupland RM, Korver A. Injuries from antipersonnel mines: the experience of the International Committee of the Red Cross. 1991;*BMJ* 1991;303:1509–12.

17 Desai MM, Zhang P, Hennessy CH. Surveillance for morbidity and mortality among older adults—United States, 1995–1996. *Morbidity & Mortality Weekly Report* 1999;48(SS-8):7–24.

18 Kannus P, Niemi S, Parkkari J, Palvanen M, Vuori I, Jarvinen M. Hip fractures in Finland between 1970 and 1997 and predictions for the future. *Lancet* 1999;353:802–5.

19 Salminen ST, Pihlajamaki HK, Avikainen VJ, Bostman OM. Population based epidemiologic and morphologic study of femoral shaft fractures. *Clin Orthop* 2000;372:241–9.

20 US Department of Health and Human Services, National Institute for Occupational Safety and Health. *Special hazard review; child labor research needs,* 1997.

21 Runyan JL. *A review of farm accident sources and research.* United States Department of Agriculture, 1993.

22 Arendt E, Dick R. Knee injury patterns among men and women in collegiate basketball and soccer. NCAA data and review of the literature. *Am J Sports Med* 1995;23:694–701.

23 Gwinn DE, Wilckens JH, McDevitt ER, Ross G, Kao TC. The relative incidence of anterior cruciate ligament injury in men and women at the United States Naval Academy. *Am J Sports Med* 2000;**28**:98–102.

24 Huston LJ, Greenfield ML, Wojtys EM. Anterior cruciate ligament injuries in the female athlete. Potential risk factors. *Clin Orthop* 2000; **372**:50–63.

25 Machold W, Kwasny O, Gabler P *et al*. Risk of injury through snowboarding. *J Trauma* 2000;**48**(6):1109–14.

26 Hunter RE. Skiing injuries. *Am J Sports Med* 1999;**27**:381–9.

27 US Department of Health and Human Services. *Musculoskeletal disorders and workplace factors. A critical review of epidemiologic evidence for work-related musculoskeletal disorders of the neck, upper extremity and low back,* 1997.

Index

Coventry University